THERAPEUTIC INTERVENTION

THERAPEUTIC INTERVENTION

Healing Strategies for Human Systems

Edited by

Uri Rueveni, Ph.D.
Clinical Associate Professor
Dept. of Psychiatry and
Human Behavior
Jefferson Medical College
Philadelphia, PA

Ross V. Speck, M.D.
Clinical Professor
Dept. of Psychiatry and Human Behavior
Jefferson Medical College
Philadelphia, PA

Joan L. Speck
Supervisor,
Family Institute
Philadelphia, PA

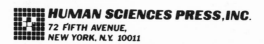

HUMAN SCIENCES PRESS,INC.
72 FIFTH AVENUE,
NEW YORK, N.Y. 10011

Copyright © 1982 by Human Sciences Press, Inc.
72 Fifth Avenue, New York, New York 10011

Printed in the United States of America
23456789   987654321

Library of Congress Cataloging in Publication Data

Main entry under title:

Therapeutic intervention.

  Includes bibliographical references and index.
  1. Social psychiatry.   2. Therapeutic community.   3. Family psychotherapy.
I. Rueveni, Uri.   II. Speck, Ross V.   III. Speck, Joan L.   [DNLM: 1. Crisis
intervention.   2. Community mental health services.   3. Family therapy.   WM 401
T398]
RC455.T52   362.2   LC 81–13501
ISBN 0–89885–086–X   AACR2

CONTENTS

CONTRIBUTORS

NANCY ANDERSON, Assistant Director of Special Education, Montgomery County Intermediate Unit, Norristown, Pennsylvania.

JOSEPH H. BERKE, M.D., Director, Arbours Association, London, England.

DAVID E. BIEGEL, L.C.S.W., Assistant Professor, School of Social Work, University of Pittsburgh, Pittsburgh, Pennsylvania.

VIVIAN GARRISON, Ph.D., Clinical Associate Professor of Psychiatry and Mental Health Services, College of Medicine and Dentistry, Newark, New Jersey.

JAMES S. GORDON, M.D., Chief, Adolescent Services Branch, Saint Elizabeth Hospital, Washington, D.C.

DENNIS T. JAFFE, Ph.D., Director, Learning for Health, Los Angeles, California.

THOMAS F. JOHNSON, Ph.D., Associate Professor, Department of Psychiatry and Human Behavior, Thomas Jefferson University, Philadelphia, Pennsylvania.

7

ROCHELLE KERN, Ph.D., Assistant Professor, Department of Sociology, New York University, New York.

ANN KLIMAN, M.A., Director, Situational Crisis Service Center for Preventive Psychiatry, White Plains, New York.

JODIE KLIMAN, Ph.D., Clinical Psychologist, Independent Practice, Cambridge, Massachusetts.

R. THOMAS MARRONE, M.D., Chief Child Psychiatrist, Montgomery County Intermediate Unit, Norristown, Pennsylvania.

ARTHUR J. NAPARSTEK, Ph.D., Director, Washington Public Affairs Center, University of Southern California, Washington, D.C.

URI RUEVENI, Ph.D., Clinical Associate Professor, Department of Psychiatry and Human Behavior, Jefferson Medical College, Thomas Jefferson University, Philadelphia, Pennsylvania.

EDMUNDO J. RUIZ, M.D., Independent Practice, Laredo, Texas.

JOANNE W. STERLING, Ph.D., Director, Bernalillo County Commmunity Mental Health/Mental Retardation Center, Albuquerque, New Mexico.

HAROLD WISE, M.D., Independent Practice; Associate Professor, Community and Preventive Medicine, Albert Einstein College of Medicine, New York, New York.

PREFACE

This is a book about interventions with people in emotional and physical crisis. Professionals in the healing fields need to conceptualize intervention approaches which can help emotionally and physically troubled people regain strength, confidence, and competence in marshalling their own as well as other people's resources available to them for coping and healing.

Most of the health and mental health delivery system approaches available today focus on the individual, with less emphasis on the family or community systems within which all of us interact. Effective models of therapeutic intervention are those which can activate the interconnectiveness of systems. Healing intervention needs to take into account the importance of linking troubled people to family, community and neighborhoods. People in trouble need to increase their participation in decision making about their lives, to marshall resources and join support groups, and to have the opportunity to develop their potential to the fullest emotionally and physically. Troubled people need to learn new skills and gain knowledge which will help them develop a sense of competence in responding to their own crisis effectively, and with the help of the resources offered them become responsible and responsive to their own process of growing and changing as all of us do.

9

Contributors to this book represent the disciplines of internal medicine, psychoanalysis, social psychiatry, child psychiatry, clinical psychology, school psychology, anthropology, and social work. Their contributions to this book were arranged in four main related intervention topics. The first is alternative services and support systems interventions (Chapters 1, 2, 3, and 4). The second series of intervention topics is on health healing (Chapters 5 and 6). The third cluster of topics discusses intervention with the family and the extended family network (Chapters 7, 8, and 9). The fourth describes crisis intervention with other systems (Chapters 10, 11, and 12).

Health professionals in the healing fields need to examine the possibility that the health and mental health delivery systems may not be functioning as effectively as they should.

Alternative services can and do provide an excellent intervention modality for many people in search of help. The variety of alternative services discussed by James Gordon in Chapter 1 is accessible and responsive to people in crisis, providing a supportive atmosphere for growth, transformation of crisis, and change.

Although alternative services are providing an important service to troubled people, the services' survival is still in question. With programs' funds being cut, what will be the future of these centers? Furthermore, what direction should the mental health delivery system take in the future? We tend to agree with James Gordon's conclusion that a change in the structure of treatment and the delivery of service is needed.

An innovative intervention is one where an anguished, frequently psychotic family member can have the opportunity to reside as a "guest" in a therapeutic community, where team efforts can reduce fears, develop trust, and heal deeply emotionally wounded persons. In Chapter 2, Joseph Berke provides us with a detailed account of his experiences with the Arbours Crisis Center, an alternative therapeutic facility located in London, England.

The dedication of the team of professionals and those committed to seeing an emotional crisis ameliorated makes the Arbours program a healing community providing an excellent alternative to hospitalization.

The practice of folk healing, a nontraditional intervention form of care-giving and counseling to troubled people, is spreading throughout the United States and the world. Mental health professionals need to take into account their clients' diverse cultural and ethnic backgrounds as well as their belief systems and rituals practiced.

In Chapter 3, Vivian Garrison provides the reader with a detailed account of one such nontraditional healing intervention, the espiritismo ritualistic folk-healing tradition, as practiced by one espiritista in

Newark's Puerto Rican community. Her documented research data direct our attention to the important roles that such practitioners play in naturally occurring support systems in various community settings.

The importance of increased awareness on the part of mental health practitioners of existing naturally occurring support systems available within one's own community and neighborhood is emphasized by Arthur Naparstek and David Biegel. Their innovative projects in two U.S. big-city neighborhoods allow the facilitation of an effective partnership between the mental health services and the community support systems.

Their mental health "capacity building model," developed through a community empowerment process, has important implications for both clinicians and mental health policy makers who need to reassess their intervention approaches with individuals and groups in different communities and neighborhoods.

We live in an era of stress and anxiety which contributes to people's emotional and physical ailments. Many new and exciting intervention programs are beginning to be developed to heal people holistically. We chose three such programs to be included in this book. In Chapter 5, Dennis Jaffe describes the development and application of the personal health exploration, a psychosocial intervention process focusing on the undertaking of a new and active role by the patients with the help of their health guide (therapist) and their physician in a process leading toward a better understanding of their disease and the crisis.

Another intervention, the therapeutic family reunion, is described by Harold Wise in Chapter 6. This healing intervention relies on the patient's own family of origin and their kin to take part in a process which can contribute to the patient's emotional and physical healing.

How can professionals develop effective intervention strategies to help families experiencing emotional crisis change? What are some of the intervention approaches available to the professional in healing the family system? In Chapter 7, Uri Rueveni describes his own framework and experience in working with families in family therapy and in family network intervention, using two strategic intervention approaches which mobilize family members to become involved in a therapeutic process of change and healing.

There are a variety of ways in which professionals can develop effective crisis intervention approaches. In Chapter 8, Edmundo Ruiz highlights the important roles various family and extended systems play in the Mexican-American culture and discusses his intervention approaches within this context.

Family therapy is the preferred modality of intervention for

Thomas Johnson who describes his work with delinquents and their family systems in Chapter 9.

An effective healing intervention is needed with people who are in prisons, or those about to be released from prisons. Do we want them to go back to lives of crime again? How can we as professionals develop some programs to help the criminal justice system intervene effectively? Efforts at a greater collaboration between the mental health system and the criminal justice system are a must if effective interventions are to take place. Some of these issues are described in Chapter 10 by Joanne Sterling who for the last ten years has been active in developing such mental health programs in Albuquerque, New Mexico.

Another difficult system in which to intervene is the school system. In Chapter 11, Nancy Anderson and Thomas Marrone describe their model of intervening in the school system, providing a variety of therapeutic services to emotionally and academically troubled students.

What are natural and human-made disasters? How can we effectively intervene? In Chapter 12, Jodie Kliman with Rochelle Kern and Ann Kliman discuss much of the published research in this area and highlight the issues and some of the ways professionals can intervene in such crisis situations.

In this book we have attempted to highlight the importance of systems concepts in dealing with human problems. It is our hope that it will broaden perspectives and further explorations in the field of human system intervention.

We want to thank our contributors for their chapter contributions, without which the ideas of this book would not have come to fruition. We also want to thank Jean Johnson who worked long and hard typing the manuscript. Finally, we want to thank our families and friends who supported us throughout the writing of this book.

Uri Rueveni
Ross V. Speck
Joan L. Speck
Philadelphia, 1982

INTRODUCTION

This book deals with interventions in healing human systems via approaches to the family system, the extended family system, the family social network, and community agencies. The mental health profession has incorporated theories and techniques garnered from diverse fields such as cybernetics (Norbert Wiener), natural history and anthropology (Gregory Bateson), and biology (Ludwig von Bertalannfy). These have all contributed to a general systems theory stratagem in attempting to solve difficult problems in living. The systems methods supplement and greatly enhance the potential to help individuals by recognizing that emotional problems frequently result from stresses outside the person in such various arenas and contexts as the family, the extended family, social class, ethnicity, or even the ecological environment.

It is interesting to note that there have been strong antagonisms between some systems theorists and some psychoanalysts. Von Bertalannfy has been accused of using machine language and metaphors (pattern, order, arrangements, mechanism, closure) and ignoring the existential person.[1] We are not polarized by this dialectic. Both theoretical stances can be useful, separately, or at times together. The world is a network of networks of systems. Von Bertalannfy recognized that living matter was hierarchically organized from the level of the atom, to the molecule, to the cell, the organ, the body, and in humans at least—the psyche, the dyad, the family, extended family, social network, network of networks, the larger society. Of course, levels have been left out of this schema, but what is important is that each level above affects and is affected by the level below. Ripples are set up which affect the entire system when a change occurs in one part of it. This can work for good or evil, for kill or cure.

A clinical example illustrates the biopsychosocial effects which ripple through a system when a change begins at one level. The family members were a 47-year-old father, a 45-year-old mother, and their 23-year-old daughter and 20-year-old son. The son had kidney failure and his mother donated a kidney for transplant. Following the surgery she became very preoccupied with her health and began to neglect her husband. The son's health improved but he and his mother seemed more symbiotically attached than prior to surgery. Father and daughter felt left out. He began dating another woman and eventually divorced his wife. The daughter left home. We do not know what other changes occurred in this family system or in the extended family. However, this type of influence at another level of a system is very common when change occurs at a different level. We could speculate in this case example that psychodynamic (psychoanalytic) factors were also at work such as oedipal attachments and fears, forcing the father to find a substitute object, as well as the daughter.

Throughout this book, the authors are suggesting a redefinition of problems and attempted solutions, taking the burden from the individual person and sharing it with a larger group of potentially supportive persons. These may be kin, friends, neighbors, or others who supply personal services, such as the hairdresser, grocer, or bartender. Support groups are made up of persons who are able to meet significant human needs by virtue of being part of an individual's social network.

The term "healing," as used in this book, does not refer to a disease in the medical sense. It emphasizes the indigenous uniqueness of a given culture or subculture and blends the nontraditional with the traditional in solving problems of physical or mental health. Much attention is paid to prevention and the individual plus the system are seen as partners in this venture.

Many human crisis situations are produced by what Alexander Leighton[2] and others have called social disintegration. These involve disruptions between persons and blood kin in particular, but also friends, neighbors, bosses, coworkers and significant others. Sudden disruptions are often labeled as crisis, while ongoing splits produce chronic stress. When the unit of observation is shifted from the individual to the social system, a whole new view of the problem and its possible alternative solutions come into focus. The labeling process itself changes.

Because psychiatry arose as a medical specialty, out of biology, physiology, and medicine, it has adopted a medical model for disturbed behavior. This medical model is aimed toward the individual whom the physician diagnoses or labels as "ill." This will determine the treatment rendered. Medicine and psychiatry have little or no nomenclature for disturbances which are interpersonal, dyadic, in the family system, or in more complex levels of society. There can be a schizophrenic label put on a person, even folie à deux (in a dyad), or maybe a "schizophrenic" society. But is a "schizophrenic" extended family or social network possible? How about a schizophrenic society or even world? What is disturbed behavior at the individual level takes on a very different hue at higher levels of social organization.

In our rapidly changing, complex, highly technological society, stress surrounds everyone. Are we to put all our mental health efforts into individual therapies, as if it is mostly or usually the individual who is the cause of breakdown? A society is much more than a sum of its individuals. Many highly complex tasks are a spin-off of cooperative efforts by many individuals.

It has been repeatedly shown that minorities, women, lower socioeconomic persons, and those undergoing culture shock have a much greater incidence of psychiatric disorder (and probably physical illness) than the general population. This is clearly a sociocultural vulnerability. This book emphasizes the importance of interventions at various societal levels, hoping to help and heal human systems as they affect the individual human being.

For this book we have asked a group of professionals in fields that are in, or allied to, the "helping" professions to suggest new and innovative ways of meeting the needs of the individual, the family, the social network, and the community within its own idiosyncratic cultural setting.

What has emerged in this endeavor is a recognition of the importance of viewing these problems—human dysfunctions—in a total context. Identity, a word much misused, is still a valid and necessary concept. It must be understood as more than an individual statement. All peoples need a sense of past, present and future. The writer, E. M. Forster, has stated that the beginning, the middle and the ending are a vital necessity to the novel, and the novel is but a reflection of the human condition at a given time and place. Without a past, mankind has no culture, without a discernible place humans have no referent, without a future we have no hope.

The segmentation of systems by modern technology, such as the mathematical gridding of a culturally recognized neighborhood into arbitrary mathematically convenient divisions, denies the membership of identity and its intrinsic singularity. By cutting across such natural boundaries, technology, in the service of convenience, abrogates the past, present, and future of the community and the identity of its personnel. As has been shown repeatedly in sociological studies, the relocation of slum societies into high-rise redevelopment projects and the concomitant stripping away of the cultural context has led to disease, destitution, and desolation—the erosion of physical, emotional, and ethical support systems.

It is to attempt a remedy for this environmental disaster—human, technological, and natural—that we have addressed this book with the hope that the interventions we have presented here will have a positive and healing effect.

Uri Rueveni
Ross V. Speck
Joan L. Speck
Philadelphia, 1982

FOOTNOTES

1. Leonard Strahl, *Conceptual Models in Psychoanalysis and the Consequences of their Application: An Epistemological Study of Philosophical-Discursive Grounds for Analytic Theories and their Clinical Implications*. Doctoral Dissertation, Heed University, Hollywood, Florida, 1980.

2. Alexander Leighton. *Social Disintegration and Mental Disorder*. Chap. 28, Vol. II, *American Handbook of Psychiatry*, 2nd edition, Silvano Arieti, Editor. New York: Basic Books, 1974.

Part I

ALTERNATIVE SERVICE AND SUPPORT SYSTEMS INTERVENTIONS

Chapter 1

ALTERNATIVE SERVICES AND MENTAL HEALTH

James S. Gordon, M.D.

With the increasing rates of alcoholism, mental breakdowns, depression, suicides, and individual and family dysfunctions, the effectiveness of the mental health delivery system is uncertain. In this chapter James Gordon claims that biomedical research does not as yet solve the pressing mental illness problems, neither are the community mental health centers able to provide effective treatment in healing people's problems.

James Gordon gives the reader an "inside feel" for the operations of the alternative services available today to help people in trouble heal themselves. A host of innovative services such as hotlines, runaway houses, crisis centers, and residential facilities for both young and old do provide an effective intervention in healing people in crisis. He concludes his chapter by looking into the future imaginatively and boldly, focusing on the concept and importance of participatory healing communities.

THE PROBLEM

Recent estimates suggest that as many as two out of 10 Americans may be in "serious need" of mental health services (Bryant, 1977). Each year almost 1% of our population is admitted to mental hospitals. And each year we consume several billion doses of Valium and Librium. Millions of people are addicted—to barbiturates, heroin, methadone, and alcohol. Psychosomatic disease is endemic. We are a people sorely troubled, desperately looking for some answer to our problems or at least some relief from them.

Too often we forget that these problems have roots in the particular conditions of our society, that any attempts to achieve "mental health" must be inseparable from efforts to create a just, decent, and personally fulfilling society. We know that poverty predisposes people to psychosis and hospitalization; that fragmenting community structures and confused family relations promote depression, alcoholism and "schizophrenia"; that pressured and alienating working conditions precipitate psychosomatic illness and drug use; that lack of employment opportunities and isolation and institutionalization depress older people. Yet we ignore this and focus our therapeutic attentions and our economic resources on individual sufferers. We call them "mentally ill," and all too often—as if their problems were simply analogous to a physical illness—treat them with drugs and electroshock treatment. When they do not get "better," we lock them up in mental hospitals.

During the last several decades the mental health establishment has adopted two major approaches to the American people's problems in living: biomedical research and the establishment of community mental health centers. Neither of them has lived up to the enthusiasm with which it was heralded. Both have been flawed by the pervasive and narrowing influence of a "medical model of mental illness."

Biomedical researchers, ignoring the total ecological context— whole people in families and communities, work places and cities— have searched for the specific anatomic locations, the physiological and biochemical causes of schizophrenia, manic depressive psychosis, depression, and anxiety. Similarly, they have experimented with medical and surgical cures—the right drug or the right operation, the right place in the brain to stimulate or depress—just as they might with treatments for diabetes or lung cancer.

The most dramatic product of early biomedical research was the development of the phenothiazine group of tranquilizers (Thorazine is the best known). Their history and their limitations are instructive. When phenothiazines were introduced in 1954 they were heralded as the "cure" for schizophrenia, the salvation of state hospital patients. An immediate exodus from state and county hospitals was followed over the years by a levelling off process. Twenty-two years later, the percentage of the overall population in mental hospitals has decreased somewhat, as has the average length of stay, but the overall numbers of patients admitted has remained about the same.

Some of those who have been "maintained" on phenothiazines, or the other still more potent drugs that were soon developed, seemed to function well outside the hospital. But many of them have come to feel as constricted, as robbed of their full potential, by the stupefying and numbing effects of the chemicals as they had been by the hospital walls. They felt as embarrassed and degraded by their dependency on powerful drugs and authoritarian doctors as they had by their reliance on prison-like institutions. Many of those who felt satisfied with the emotional level on which their medication kept them have found themselves experiencing severe physical "side effects"—impotence, extreme sensitivity to sunlight, chronic skin rashes, easy tiring, obesity, and the chronic, often irreversible debilitating neurological disorder, tardive dyskinesia.

The passage of the Community Mental Health Centers Act in 1963 was to be an even more important milestone. Hailed as a "bold new approach" by John F. Kennedy, it signalled a modification of the medical model, a growing sensitivity to the effects of poverty and social stress on the creation of "mental illness"; an increasing awareness of the possibilities of helping people to change by working with them, their families, and their communities to change their social situation. Community mental health centers were designed to help prevent institutionalization; to bring low cost, readily available mental health services, including individual and group psychotherapy, to large numbers of people; and to make—through "consultation and education"—changes in families, schools, and communities which would forestall the development of mental illness in their members.

In fact, the community mental health centers have never resolved the contradiction between a social and a medical definition of "mental illness." Their legislative mandate depends on their responsiveness to community needs, on their capacity for helping people not to become chronic mental patients, and, ultimately, on their ability to change those conditions which make people "mentally ill." But the political power, social prestige, professional status and high incomes of their leaders come from their roles as doctors and mental health professionals. Too many community mental health centers simply perpetuate the medical model and in so doing provide inappropriate services.

In outpatient clinics that are little more than an aggregation of private therapists' offices, they may insist that people fit into one or another diagnostic category and predetermined therapeutic experience. Instead of providing the services—economic and educational, vocational, and counseling—that are necessary to help seriously disturbed people live successfully at home and in their community, they tend to obliterate anxiety about these problems with maintenance doses of antidepressants and phenothiazines. The consultation and education that they provide is often directed at strengthening the skills of other professionals—teachers, guidance counselors, etc.—rather than, say, changing the classroom conditions which frustrate students, teachers, and guidance counselors alike. Rarely do they provide services to people who, though needy, are unwilling to define and stigmatize themselves as mentally ill. Still more rarely do staff members spend substantial amounts of time in the community they are supposed to serve.

All during my medical and psychiatric training I was deeply troubled by the institutional condescension and coercion with which the medical model was compounded—enforced medication, electroshock treatment, locked doors, and seclusion rooms—and by the narrowness to which it urged its adherents.

Doing psychotherapy with poor people in a community mental health center I became increasingly sensitive to the wrongheadedness of an ideology which emphasized talking about intrapsychic difficulties and largely ignored the day-to-day realities which confronted people when, after an hour, they left my office. I discovered how much faster some of the most troubled people would lose their "psychotic symptoms," if I devoted more of my energy to understanding the concrete and oppressive realities of their lives—and then helped them deal with those realities.

Driving one man to a welfare office; waiting with him; helping him prod its sluggish and indifferent bureaucracy into giving him emergency payments let him know more graphically than any words that I really did "care" about him. Afterward he spoke much more easily of his "personal" problems.

Visiting a "paranoid" teenager in her home, I discovered that her parents *were* constantly invading and intruding—on her room, her mail, her bureau drawers, her phone calls, even the pockets of her blue jeans. I obviously had to take her seriously when she told me that "they're as crazy as I am." She could not possibly become less "paranoid" until they changed.

Working with a "Crisis Intervention Team" in the psychiatric emergency room of a municipal hospital I discovered that the vast majority of those who would have otherwise been admitted could be helped to stay at home. With the intensive involvement of the crisis team (a psychologist, a nurse, and three paraprofessionals) a family could pull together to help one of its members during a psychotic episode or suicidal depression. While they assisted family members in dealing with external problems (welfare, job, housing, food), the team used the crisis as a lever to help them understand the particular dynamics which had precipitated it. Often, in a few weeks, without hospitalizing anyone, they were to help a family resolve a situation which had seemed intolerable.

During the time that I was in charge of a hospital ward I discovered how much "better" off psychotic patients—and staff—could be, if they were simply treated with the respect due other human beings. In the context of a community in which they were given power over their own lives, in which they took part in making rules and in working out cooperative living arrangements, a group of "mental patients" simply stopped being so disturbed. Given trust, or at least the possibility of it, by a staff that refused to characterize their speech and behavior as symptomatology, the patients were often able to trust and get help from staff members; free to come and go, they tended to stay and try to work out their problems; allowed to regulate their own medication they tended to use it occasionally, when necessary, and to avoid becoming dependent on it. "Everywhere else" one "chronic schizophrenic" young man told me, "I'm crazy; here I'm sane."

Still, I concluded that the reforms that could be made within the context of traditional mental health settings, were severely limited by the structure of those settings, and by the ideology of mental illness to which the professionals who dominate them subscribe. When I entered the U.S. Public Health Service, I decided to look for places in which troubled people could be helped—and could help themselves—without so many constraints.

Alternative Services

Six years ago I began to work as consultant, researcher, and colleague with "alternative human services." I wanted to see if the ideology of professionalism really did make it more difficult to meet the needs of some troubled people; if changing the setting in which help was given and the set of those who were giving it made a substantial difference in the people who received it; if some of the culturally alien but side-effect-free techniques they were using with their clients—meditation, massage, acupressure—might contribute to promoting their well-being; and if the skills I had developed in my psychiatric training could be effectively shared with and enlarged by groups of dedicated nonprofessionals. I am still working with alternative services. I do not think they have "the answer" to people's problems in living, but they are surely dealing with them in a way that is respectful, open minded, and effective.

Alternative services are approximately ten years old. Most of the early ones were founded by indigenous helpers, in direct response to the physical and emotional needs of the disaffected young people who in the mid- to late-1960s migrated to their communities as alternatives to health, mental health, and social service facilities which the young found threatening, demeaning, or unresponsive.

The founders of the first alternative services resembled the earlier settlement house workers in their idealism and humanitarianism. They differed in their commitment to the kind of participatory democracy which animated the civil rights, antiwar, youth, and women's movements of the 1960s (Gordon, 1974). These activist workers believed that, given time and space to do it, ordinary people could help themselves and one another to deal with the vast majority of problems in living that confronted them. They questioned the appropriateness of professional services which labeled or stigmatized those who came for help, and, in their own work, blurred or obliterated boundaries between staff and clients; e.g., a teenager who was panicky one night might counsel another the next. Determined to remain responsive to their clients' needs, these early workers continually advocated the social changes that would make individual change more possible.

In 1967, a handful of switchboards, drop-in centers, free clinics, and runaway houses served marginal young people in the "hip" neighborhoods of a few large cities. Today there are approximately 2000 hotlines, over 200 runaway houses, and 400 free clinics. They have been organized by people of all ages, classes, and ideologies in small towns, suburbs, and rural areas, as well as in the large cities. In Prince George county, a suburban and rural Maryland county, for example, one of three hotlines receives 1400 calls a month, one of two runaway houses gives shelter and intensive counseling to over 350 young people each year, and a single one of the county's nine drop-in centers provides 600 hours of individual therapy each month (Gordon, 1978a).

In the early years, alternative services were preoccupied with responding to the immediate needs of their young clients—for emergency medical care, a safe place during a bad drug trip, or short-term housing. More recently, they have expanded and diversified. Drop-in centers work with the families and teachers of the teenagers who come to them as well as the young people themselves. Runaway houses have opened long-term residences and foster-care programs for those who cannot return home or would otherwise be institutionalized; and free clinics and hotlines have helped to start specialized counseling services for other and older groups such as women, gays, the elderly, etc.

In the 1970s, the alternative service model has been adopted by people who have identified new community needs. They have created drug and alcohol counseling programs, rape crisis centers, shelters for battered women, peer counseling and street work projects, holistic health centers, home birthing services, and programs designed specifically for old people and particular ethnic minorities.

Many of these programs are beginning to emphasize the role of diet, exercise, and lifestyle in precipitating and preventing physical and emotional dysfunction and the relationship between stress and physical and emotional illness. Some are using the centuries-old preventive medical techniques of Chinese medicine, of yoga and herbalism, of homeopathy, massage, and chiropractic, and such modern self-help techniques as biofeedback, guided imagery, and lifestyle counseling to help their clients to achieve physical and emotional balance. Increasingly, workers in alternative services are regarding these and other psychophysical techniques as a natural complement to a system of care which emphasizes the whole person in a supportive environment, the ability of people to help themselves and one another.

CHARACTERISTICS OF ALTERNATIVE SERVICES

Though alternative services are as diverse in their operation, staff, and structure as their communities and clients, they share certain philosophical assumptions, attitudes, and practices which define their approach to mental health and illness as "alternative" and make them particularly useful and responsive to the people they serve. I have found the following to be among the most significant:

They respond to people's problems as those problems are experienced. A woman whose husband is beating her is regarded as a victim, not scrutinized as a masochist. A child who leaves his home is seen, housed, and fed as a runaway, not diagnosed as an "acting out disorder" or judged as a "status offender." A man with chronic back pain and no demonstrable organic lesion is treated as a sufferer not dismissed as a "psycho" or a "crock."

They provide services that are immediately accessible with a minimum of waiting and bureaucratic restriction. Hotlines, shelters for battered women, rape crisis centers, runaway houses and many drop-in centers are open twenty-four hours a day, free, to anyone who calls or comes in off the street.

They tend to treat their clients' problems as signs of change and opportunities for growth rather than symptoms of an illness which must be suppressed. In drug-free alternatives to mental hospitalization like Diabasis and Soteria, even psychotic episodes are regarded as potentially transformative and illuminating experiences.

They treat those who come to them for help as members of families and social systems. This enables them to view their troubled clients' "symptoms" as reactions to and communications within their familial or social situation. It provides the underpinning for their treatment of pregnancy, childbirth, and dying primarily as shared family experiences and only secondarily, and occasionally, as medical conditions or emergencies. On a programmatic level this "systems" viewpoint encourages many alternative services to advocate for and work with their clients in the arena—job, home, school, or court—in which their problems arise.

They make use of mental health professionals and the techniques they have developed but depend on nonprofessionals to deliver most of the primary care. In projects as diverse as runaway houses and home birth programs, free clinics and alternatives to mental hospitalization professionals serve almost exclusively as consultants, trainers, and emergency backup. They are there to share their knowledge with staff and clients and not necessarily to run the service.

They regard active client participation as the cornerstone of their mental health service program and indeed of mental health. On an individual therapeutic level this means emphasizing the strength of those who seek help and their capacity for self-help. Teenage runaways are encouraged to see themselves as potential agents for a family's change rather than helpless victims of its oppression; battered wives to become strong enough to leave rather than endure their husbands' brutality. In dozens of "humanistic gerontology" programs and in hundreds of free clinics and holistic healing centers, clients are encouraged to use techniques like biofeedback, progressive relaxation, acupressure, and guided imagery, and disciplines like Yoga and Tai Chi to experience, and then alter, physical and emotional states that they had always regarded as beyond their control.

On an organizational level, this emphasis on self-help leads most alternative services to include present and former clients in their decision-making structure. It means devoting time and energy to creating formal and informal ways for those who have been helped to use their personal experience as a basis for helping others.

They provide both clients and staff with a supportive and enduring community which transcends the delivery or receipt of a particular service. In a time when the extended family is losing its coherence and ties to hometowns and neighborhoods are fraying, alternative services are providing a continuing focus for collective allegiance and an opportunity for long-term mutual support. For many who have long ago ceased to be official clients or workers they remain a retreat in times of trouble and a place to gather to celebrate joyous occasions.

They can provide care that is by any standards equal or superior to that offered by traditional mental health services. Many of the reports are anecdotal (i.e., the consistent finding that large numbers of young people with psychotic or borderline diagnoses are diverted from hospitalization by a variety of alternative services), but "harder" data are also beginning to accumulate. A two-year follow-up study of Sotería, a National Institute of Mental Health funded residential alternative to hospitalization, revealed that residents of the program "showed significantly better occupational levels and were more able to leave home to live independent of their families of origin" than a control group of people hospitalized in a crisis-oriented general hospital ward (Mosher and Menn, 1977); evaluation of the S.A.G.E. (Senior Actualization and

Growth Explorations) project in Berkeley has revealed striking psychological, cognitive, and physical improvements in the older people who participated in the program of gentle physical exercise, meditation, and group discussion (Lieberman, 1978); and a matched population study of 1046 home births and 1046 hospital births has revealed significantly more infections and birth injuries in the group of babies that was delivered in the hospital (Mehl, 1977).

They are in general more economical than the traditional services which their clients might otherwise use. Young people, many of whom come to runaway centers to avoid being hospitalized, provide an interesting example: In 1975, an NIMH study of 15 runaway centers around the country revealed that runaway centers spent from $32 to 50 a day for each young person housed; in contrast, the figures for acute care hospitalization ranged from $125 to 200 a day (Gordon, 1975). A more recent and sophisticated analysis of one runaway house, Someplace Else, in Tallahassee, Florida, revealed that this program was approximately three times as cost effective as the services routinely offered by the county. Long-term residential alternatives to hospitalization for adults like Sotería and the Training in Community Living program of the Mendota Mental Health Institute tend to be more expensive but here too cost benefit analysis seems to reveal significant advantages for the alternative services (Weisbrod, 1977).

They have financial problems. The desire to work with whoever comes to them regardless of economic compensation; their attempts to provide comprehensive and often unreimbursed services; their unwillingness to take funds which restrict their work with clients; the complexity of federal, state, and local funding procedures; and the general reluctance of many agencies to fund service programs that are neither certified by a professional establishment nor proven in "scientific terms" all conspire to keep most alternative services chronically underfunded.

They use their experience in trying to meet people's direct service needs as a basis for advocacy efforts on their clients' behalf. Hotlines which have noted an increase in a particular kind of problem—battered women, child abuse, etc.—have used their statistical information and their moral authority as service providers to prod local mental health and social service agencies to create programs to meet these needs. Groups which serve old people, pregnant women and runaways have organized on a state and national level to advocate legislation and funding to further and protect their clients' interests.

They regard it as their responsibility to change and expand the work they do to meet the changing needs of their clients. During the last several years, for example, centers for runaways have enlisted professionals to help them create family counseling programs. They have opened long-term residences and foster-placement programs for young people who cannot or will not go home; drop-in centers for teenagers who are having problems at home but do not want to leave their families; and educational, vocational, and health care services to equip all these young people to survive and deal with the adult world.

PROSPECTS FOR THE FUTURE

Many alternative services combine the skills and thoroughness of professionals with the commitment to service, responsiveness, and organizational flexibility of nonprofessionals. They are already providing effective, low cost mental health services to large numbers— probably several millions—of Americans of all ages, races, and classes (Gordon, 1978b). Any attempt to make mental health services more responsive to people's felt needs should take account of the kinds of programmatic innovations that alternative services have been making, of the new techniques being developed in holistic health practice, and of the spirit which pervades the entire alternative service movement.

Though some alternative services will function best when dealing with a particular problem or group, others may in the future evolve into new kinds of central places where troubled and troubling people could be offered comprehensive services. These new places could continue to be called community mental health centers, but they might better be called "human service centers" or "community centers" or simply "centers." The names, designed to indicate a responsiveness to people's needs, would avoid creating the feelings of deprecation inevitably associated with describing oneself as "mentally ill."

Instead of spending the majority of their time seeing patients in their offices, professionals in these centers would largely devote themselves to a much expanded version of the "consultation and education" that is now so often neglected. Their primary job would be to consult with community people about the services they have already begun, and to catalyze, but not dominate, efforts to create new residential, counseling, and community development programs.

Rather than define problems in mental health terminology, center staff would help people to define their own problems in their own terms. If a woman with five children were suicidally depressed because of the inadequacy of her welfare payments, the dreariness of her home, and the rats that threaten her family, the center's crisis team would work first of all on these realities, and help her deal with the welfare department, assist her with child care, and bring in an exterminator. Instead of involving her in long-term psychotherapy or drug treatment, it might help her become part of a support group of parents in similar situations. In the context of this group she might at some point feel free to talk about the "personal problems" which so many mental health professionals would insist on "attacking" first.

For people who needed them, various kinds of residences would be available. Thus, someone experiencing the personality disintegration and overwhelming anxiety that often signal an acute psychotic episode would be able to go to a crisis house or to stay with a family where he could be guided and protected by a specially patient and skillful staff. There symptoms would not be suppressed by drugs. Instead, the psychotic episode could become the kind of natural healing process that it is in some traditional societies and in such modern experimental communities as California's Soteria and Diabasis. Similarly, center workers might consult with or help start shelters for other groups—young people who could not live at home, or "women in transition," or older individuals without social support—where these people could gain perspective on their lives and share their problems without defining themselves as mentally ill.

Though a dangerous and uncontrollable few would continue to require institutionalization, the vast majority of those who need longer-term care could be kept in their own communities in ordinary houses easily accessible to friends and relatives. Many of these people could, if staff workers provided organization and leadership, learn to take care of one another. Already some shelters for battered women and residences for older teenagers are run by clients; certainly old people who are healthy but homeless could supervise the care of young people who are chronically ill; and students at colleges or young workers could be subsidized—well below the cost of conventional foster care—to live with runaways who lack homes to return to.

The majority of people with problems do not, of course, need crisis intervention or residential services. Instead of assuming they needed "therapy," centers would offer them the resources—professional expertise, advocacy, and education—to help them deal with their own problems. People would be helped to understand themselves as participants in and often enough sufferers from the concrete situations of their life—a part of a family, an office, a work group or a class. Techniques of family counseling, group therapy, and community organizing could be used to help make the family, the classroom, or the work place more responsive to all of its participants, to give them the tools to continue to work things out long after the center workers withdraw.

At the same time, some centers might begin to provide the kind of ongoing individualized health care which has been lacking in our society. Under the supervision of physicians who are developing a holistic perspective on health and mental health, physician's assistants, nurse practitioners, and neighborhood people trained by them could discuss and review each person's physical and emotional well-being, could investigate the economic, occupational, familial, and intra-psychic causes of stress in their lives. Together they could formulate a regime of diet, exercise, and relaxation, or help them to look for other employment, more education, or different housing.

Groups of people with special concerns or problems—women wanting to share with each other questions about their roles as women; parents of retarded or autistic children, old people wishing to improve their psychological and physical functioning—would be helped, if needed, to form groups with or without a leader in which they could discuss and deal with their common concerns.

Individual therapy would still be available, but there would be a shift in emphasis toward helping people to develop the capacity to analyze their social situations and physical and emotional needs and thus be able to use a network of helpers both within the center and outside. The original aspect of this treatment would also change. Instead of relying on drugs to elevate mood or calm anxiety, to deaden headaches or stop gastric secretion, people would be taught to deal with these conditions through biofeedback, meditation, yoga, acupressure, Tai Chi, and massage. Learning to use these "self-help" techniques would enable people to avoid prolonged dependency on professional helpers; contribute to their sense of control over their own lives; and remove the possibility of dangerous side effects and diminished performance which always attend the use of psychotropic drugs.

This kind of center could be a continuing source of the kinds of "primary prevention" programs that the mental health establishment often talks of but rarely spends time and money to bring about. Together, staff and clients of the center could help other agencies develop education, recreation, and community-action programs, and campaign for more responsive policies in the institutions which affect people's lives, from welfare offices to hospitals to factories. For the community as a whole, the center—which would have clients on its governing board—would be the kind of gathering place that alternative services already are, a place where people could come when they wanted to help as well as be helped, when they just felt like being with others, as well as when they were in trouble.

Any attempt to make the kinds of changes that I have described will require a different attitude, a new kind of training—not only of the physicians, psychologists, and social workers who will help facilitate this change but of the paraprofessionals and the clients with whom they will work. Professionals need training which helps them to understand how their attitudes and convictions are formed by their own values and culture, and how these may at times prevent them from working effectively with people. They need to learn also that in addition to being bearers of knowledge and purveyors of new techniques they are the servants of those for whom they work. At the same time, community people who crave a common purpose and some larger goal will have the opportunity to learn and use new skills.

In the context of a participatory healing community the boundaries between helpers and helped will blur and the very nature of mental health work will be transformed. Even the most arduous tasks may well change their character: For most attendants the experience of working with mad people in a hospital setting is grim, demeaning, and uncomfortable; working with the same people in a place like Soteria or Diabasis or in one of the group foster homes that I have helped develop is, though exhausting, enormously exciting and challenging.

The point of all this is not simply to produce another kind of treatment, or another kind of professional, and certainly not to insist that all centers do all things in a particular way; but to change the structure of treatment and the delivery of services; to relate to troubled people on their terms; to insist that their needs—not the preconceptions or self interest of any professional group—shape the kind of help they receive; to give them the opportunity to use their full potential and to heal themselves; and to support and enlarge—not usurp—the kinds of initiatives that alternative services have already taken. None of the reforms I have proposed is utopian—and all of them together will not of course create a utopia, but they are a start, a step toward relieving at least some of the human misery that we have too complacently and too long regarded as the symptoms of mental illness.

References

Bryant, T. *Preliminary Report of the President's Commission on Mental Health.* HEW, Washington, D.C. September, 1977.

Gordon, J. S. Coming together: Consultation with young people. *Social Policy,* 1974.

Gordon, J. S. Alternative services: A recommendation for public funding. 1975 (unpublished).

Gordon, J. S. Statistics gathered by the Special Study on Alternative Services for the President's Commission on Mental Health. 1978a. HEW, Washington, D.C.

Gordon, J. S. Final report of the Special Study on Alternative Services to the President's Commission on Mental Health, 1978b. HEW Washington, D.C.

Lieberman, M. Personal communication.

Mehl, L. E. Research on alternatives in childbirth: What can it tell us about hospital practice. *Twenty-first Century Obstetrics,* National Association of Parents and Professionals for Safe Alternatives in Childbirth, 1977.

Mosher, L. R., and Menn, A. Z. Community residential treatment for schizophrenia: Two year follow-up data. 1977 (unpublished).

Weisbrod, B. A., Test, M. A., and Stein, L. I. An alternative to the mental hospital benefits and cost. 1977 (unpublished).

Chapter 2

AN ALTERNATIVE SANCTUARY

The Arbours Crisis Center
Joseph H. Berke, M.D.

The Arbours Crisis Center offers a wide range of interventions with individuals, couples, families, and social networks as an alternative to hospitalization and frequently as an alternative to medication. The Arbours Center is complemented by and is part of a network of therapists and facilities including three long-stay therapeutic communities. Humanitarian factors, flexibility, and common sense govern the choice of therapeutic, usually psychotherapeutic, services provided. This chapter by Joseph Berke offers several detailed examples with outcomes.

The Arbours Association was established in 1970 by Dr. Morton Schatzman, myself, and others in order to help people in emotional distress and as an alternative to mental hospitals. The Arbours sponsors three long-stay therapeutic communities, a training program in psychotherapy, and a psychotherapy clinic.

In 1973 we set up the Arbours Crisis Center in order to provide immediate and intensive personal support and accommodation for individuals, couples or families threatened by sudden mental and social breakdown. This happens when people find that they cannot cope with life's ordinary as well as extraordinary demands. These difficulties may be developmental—adolescence, menopause, old age—situational, e.g., moving, entering school, hospitalization, or interpersonal, e.g., marriage, divorce, or the death of a friend or relative. In response, people describe a constellation of feelings including anxiety, guilt, fear, confusion, and depression. Moreover, marked changes in behavior and habits may accompany a pervasive helplessness and hopelessness.

These crises are turning points leading to collapse and chaos or to personal growth and development. What happens not only depends on the person in crisis, but on the attitudes of friends, family and whomever he or she has turned to for help. All too often these people are frightened by the emotional turmoil that accompanies and is part of the crisis. Then the whole event is likely to be seen as a sign of mental illness, as a "disease" which must be treated and stopped, rather than as an expression of disease which should be tolerated, and can be eased, if not alleviated by understanding and practical support. Whatever is done, it is important to avoid cultural *closure*. This is a term and concept developed by the British psychiatrist, Dr. R. D. Scott. *Cultural closure* is the moment when one member of a family is no longer seen and accepted as part of the family, but as a stranger, alienated from and by the family (or group, or society). *Closure* accompanies diagnosis, a process of invalidation whereby a man or woman is deemed "in-valid," a mental "invalid" stripped of responsibility for his thoughts, feelings or actions.[1] Dr. Scott points out that once this has occurred, and the exfamily member has been sent for treatment, it is very difficult for him or her to regain his prior identity or standing in the family or community. A major purpose of the Arbours Crisis Center is to provide as much support as necessary, not only to the person in crisis, but to his whole family or social network, so that *closure* can be avoided.

The Arbours Center is a substantial, semi-detached house located in a quiet, residential neighborhood of North London. Three psychotherapists live at the Center. They are assisted by a resource group of psychotherapists, doctors, social workers, and trainees.

The Center answers several dozen calls or letters a week from people in all walks of life and with all sorts of problems. Often callers seem to need no more than a short opportunity to speak with another human being who is sympathetic, tolerant, and willing to absorb some of their distress. On other occassions, the calls may be extended phone consultations lasting upward of an hour and a half. In either case these examples of brief psychotherapy may be repeated two or more times before the caller calms down and the immediate upset is resolved. David Stafford, currently resident therapist at the Center, has described one such intervention:

It was a Sunday afternoon about 5:30. I received a call from a panic-stricken lady who was worried about feeling strange and tense. I asked her what this was about. She didn't know but said that her feelings were so overwhelming that she might explode. I asked her about her living arrangements. She said she had been divorced for two years. Her teenaged daughter had been living with her exhusband, but they had had a row and she had recently returned home. This situation had not been working out well. The relationship was quite strained, but the woman had not been able to discuss this with anyone.

I suggested that her strange feelings had to do with her daughter, that she was full of pent-up anger because her daughter had chosen to live with her father in the first place, but that she had never talked to her daughter about this.

The woman replied in a surprised tone of voice that I was right. She said she had been furious both with her daughter and her exhusband. On the other hand she was glad that her daughter had returned and hoped she would stay.

I suggested that she probably hadn't told her daughter how angry she felt because she was frightened her daughter would leave.

The caller agreed and we continued to talk about this for another five or ten minutes. By now she was calmer and she told me that she was feeling much better. She said she was tired and wanted to go to sleep. I thought this was a good idea and asked her to call me back later on and let me know how things were. She was pleased with my suggestion.

About 11:00 P.M. she called back and said she had had a good sleep. She had dreamed a lot about her childhood. She also mentioned that her daughter had gone out to a disco but should be back soon. I asked her if she thought she could discuss some of her feelings with her daughter. She didn't think so, but agreed to call back in the morning and let me know.

About 10:30 the following morning she called back. The woman was a bit anxious. She had discussed things with her daughter and had been surprised to learn that her daughter had also felt angry and guilty. After a brief further discussion I gave her the number of our psychotherapy clinic. I also told her she was free to call back if she wished.

Later in the day I received one last call from her. The woman was still a bit anxious, but she generally felt better because things were clearer for her. She thanked me for my time and support.

This phone service is one of the most active aspects of the work of the Center. It is funded entirely by the Arbour Association which is a registered charity.[2] Obviously, not all calls are resolved so quickly. After speaking with the caller, the resident therapist may decide that a personal consultation would be useful, or the caller may request it. Then we try to arrange an appointment within 24 hours. We tell the caller that a team of therapists from the Center will be meeting him, and others involved in the crisis.

The crisis team consists of the team leader, a resident therapist, and a member of the Arbours training program. The team leader is an experienced psychiatrist or psychotherapist whose function is to assist in the evaluation of the crisis and to coordinate the efforts of the team on behalf of the person or persons in difficulty.

We prefer to make the initial consultation at the home of the caller or of the person who is allegedly in crisis. Home visits are a much better source of information about people and relationships than a multitude of meetings with single family members outside the home. The team makes this initial visit without prior assumptions about who is "mad" or who is "ill." The purpose of the meeting is to try to find out who is in crisis, who is affected by the crisis (and who is affecting it) and what the crisis is about. This is not a straightforward task, because people tend to hide what is bothering them even when they are most desperately asking for help.

Interestingly, the most overtly disturbed members of a family or group are not necessarily the ones in greatest crisis, or, from their point of view, in crisis at all. It often transpires that the person making the initial approach to the Center is in crisis, no matter how upset or frankly psychotic others in the family may be.[3]

On one occasion we received a call from a nurse on behalf of a friend, a divorcee, who lived alone with her young daughter. The nurse was very anxious because her friend had not eaten for several days, had been having frequent nightmares, and had been neglecting her daughter and herself. I was the leader of the team that went to visit the woman in her home. When we arrived, we discovered that the woman was asleep in bed and did not want to be disturbed. The daughter had been sent to her grandparents. The nurse was there with several people, all of whom were very upset. They had been trying to care for the woman for three days and felt they could do no more. They were preparing to send her to a mental hospital.

So our first discovery was that the person allegedly in crisis was asleep and that everyone else was at crisis point. Moreover, the helpers proposed to deal with their crisis by sending the sleeping lady away for treatment which she did not want. How had all this developed? It transpired that the woman and her friends all dabbled in the occult. In fact, she was quite well known as a reader of palms. When she became upset, her friends decided that she had become possessed by a bad spirit. The nurse was convinced that exorcism was the sole answer. Had she ever exorcised a bad spirit before? Oh no, but she did not think it was too difficult. She had seen it done before, in the movies. So she had laid out some candles and begun chanting. Further questions revealed that there was a connection between the ceremonials and the nightmares, the more of one, the more of the other. The nurse had not appreciated this. She had become very upset when her exorcism had not eliminated the bad spirits, and had redoubled her efforts.

Tactfully, I pointed out that exorcism is a very skilled business. Perhaps she did not have sufficient expertise to conquer the spirits in question. The nurse agreed. I also observed that everyone seemed tired and could use a good night's sleep. So the nurse went home, and the others prepared some food for the palm reader who, by now, had woken up and was darting in and out of the sitting room. She wanted to know what had been going on.

Soon afterward, my colleagues and I left too, but not before letting everyone know that they could call us as needed. Days later we received a grateful call from the nurse. Her friend had calmed down and had returned to reading palms. She herself was back at work and had decided to refrain from exorcism for the foreseeable future.

Many callers have made up their mind in advance of meeting with us that one or more members of their family should come to the Center. This indicates the tremendous anxiety that has been aroused and that *closure* has or is about to occur. On another occasion a young woman called the Center on behalf of her fiancé. He had not slept for a week, was talking in a strange tongue and was obsessed with Egyptian gods and godesses. Not only was she exhausted but the young man's family were thinking of having him committed. Could he please come to the Center immediately.

Our first task was to calm and reassure the caller. She seemed close to breaking point herself because of her attempts to help her boyfriend. We gently said that it might be possible for the man to come to the Center, if he wished, but to begin we preferred to visit him at home. I was a part of the team that made the initial visit.

It turned out that the young man had just retired as a dope dealer. Previously he had made a lot of money and, in certain circles, was a powerful and influential person. Now he was unsure of himself. He did not know what to do with his life and was quite depressed. But he denied this by bullying his friends and family into believing that he had special and magical powers. Clinically his behavior could be termed "manic."

At first he did not want to see us because he was frightened that I would say he was "mad." Actually, he was quite aware of what was going on, but he had boxed himself into an untenable position both with himself and his friends. He thought that if he revealed he was not all powerful, then he would lose face with his friends and would be ignored by them. Yet the more domineering and omnipotent he tried to appear, the more he was assailed by evidence that he was small and unimportant. In order to blot out this evidence, he forced himself to get "high," and ever "higher" and "higher."

It did not take him long to appreciate that I had not come to take him away, neither to declare him insane, nor to take the side of his family against him. Similarly, it did not take him long to discover that he could not bully me and that I was not frightened by incense, hieroglyphics, or magic spells. Once these preliminaries were out of the way we had rather a good talk about what really concerned him and the difficulties he faced. Then he calmed down and so did everyone else. We all agreed that he did not need to come to the Center, but left it open for him or his family to keep in touch with the Center. The young man and his fiancée decided to go on holiday for a few weeks. Upon his return I saw him for two consultations. He was out of dope, out of Egypt, and making plans to go straight.

There are times when it is helpful for the person or persons in crisis to move to the Center. This happens when they have been living alone and cannot cope with the day-to-day running of their lives, when their family or friends cannot cope, or when there is so much hostility between them and others that a period of separation is necessary in order to ease the antagonism and tension. The Arbours Crisis Center is the only facility that I know that will give shelter and support to an entire family on short notice, including the family pet. I have described one such intervention with Tony, a very depressed musician, in a previous book (Berke, 1979). He only agreed to come to the Center if his wife and child and best friend and pet beagle could come too. We were amused that when Tony and his family went home, the beagle wished to stay.

People who stay at the Center are often very depressed, very anxious, or psychotic. The usual boundaries that exist between them and others, between animate and inanimate, may have become blurred, or broken down entirely. As a rule the more difficult the intervention, the more we call on other therapists working at the Center to join the team. Our object is not simply to stop bizarre or disruptive experience or behavior, but to contain it and make sense of it. These goals are interconnected. Our guests need help because they are no longer able to keep in themselves, and to themselves, wildly distressing thoughts, feelings, and wishes. The Center, both the building and the therapists, provide this help by serving as temporary containers for intolerable fear and rage, confusion, and criticism. This process is akin to what passes between parents and children, when the children scream and cry, and the mother and father hold and absorb these screams and tears and make the world bearable again.

This process of containment is an essential component of psychotherapy. The British psychoanalyst, Dr. Hanna Segal (1975), has linked what happens in therapy to what goes on between mother and infant:

> When an infant has an intolerable anxiety, he deals with it by projecting it into the mother. The mother's response is to acknowledge this anxiety and do whatever is necessary to relieve the infant's distress. The infant's perception is that he has projected something intolerable into his object, but the object was capable of containing it and dealing with it. He can then reintroject not only the original anxiety, but an anxiety modified by having been contained. He also reintrojects an object capable of containing and dealing with anxiety. The containment of the anxiety by an internal object capable of understanding is the beginning of mental stability.

We make things bearable again by tolerating the pain and discomfort in ourselves, by suffering on behalf of another. Concomitantly we try to evaluate and understand what the distress is about. We seek to digest and assimilate the very experiences which, to our guests, appear crazy, unintelligible, dangerous and indigestible. By feeding our understanding back, gently, slowly, we help them to make links between what they have been feeling and what has been going on in their lives. Then they can regain and contain their experiences and a sense of their integrity and autonomy. In other words, our task is to perceive and apperceive on behalf of our guests, to enable them to face reality and to dream.

The process of digesting the seemingly indigestible is another essential component of psychotherapy. It has been described by the British psychoanalyst, Dr. Wilfred R. Bion (1977) in his book, *Learning from Experience*. He calls the indigestible bits, "beta elements." These are concrete sense impressions, not amenable to use in dream thought but suitable for projective identification. They are influential in acting out. They are objects that can be evacuated or used for a kind of thinking that depends on the manipulation of what are felt to be things in themselves as if to substitute such manipulation for words or ideas.

"Beta elements" can be transformed into "alpha elements" which are digestible and symbolic, the necessary components of thinking, understanding, dreaming, and remembering. Maturation is the process of such transformation.

It may be said that during a crisis, the person(s) in severe distress regresses to the point where "beta elements" and beta functioning predominate. The purpose of the crisis intervention is to help the person(s) concerned by tolerating his "beta elements" and then facilitating the reemergence of "alpha functioning."

During the course of our interventions we may spend a great deal of time with our guests and members of their family, or not. Some guests prefer to be left more to themselves. We may do a lot of interpretive work, or very little. We aim to establish a supportive relationship without becoming intrusive and overbearing. Every guest attends two or more team meetings a week lasting from one to four hours. There are many more informal discussions with the resident therapists. Our orientation is psychodynamic. Some of the team leaders prefer to work primarily with and through the family, or social network. Others, like myself, emphasize an intensive psychoanalytic psychotherapy. In either case we endeavor to avoid medication because this diminishes the capacity of people to come to grips with their emotional and mental state and to work through feelings which may be at the root of their difficulties. Obviously when a person has taken psychotropic drugs for long periods and has become dependent on them, or is in such emotional pain that he or she requests a tranquilizer, we concur. This is an infrequent occurrence. More commonly people ask us to help them diminish or stop taking previously prescribed and usually excessive amounts of tranquilizers (phenothiazines) or antidepressants.[4]

It should be obvious from my brief description of several interventions that a crisis rarely involves a single person. On the contrary the mental and social disequilibrium that results when one member of a family or social network reaches a developmental, situational or interpersonal turning point reverberates throughout his or her relationships. These reverberations themselves can be considered mini-crises, or foci of disequilibrium that threaten other relatives and friends, if not the whole network, itself. For the crisis to pass and for a new equilibrium to be established it is often necessary to support everyone in the network, not just the person most overtly disturbed. With this in mind, I shall now describe an intervention we made on behalf of a man who had become acutely psychotic while on a visit to London with his wife.

I shall call this couple Peter and Susan Atkins. Both are in their 40s and came from the north of England. He is a businessman and she is a scriptwriter for television. One Sunday morning I received a call from Mrs. Atkins. She was worried about her husband who had become very distraught after posting a notice about nuclear war on the wall of a public library. For several days he had been wildly demanding like a baby, as well as withdrawn and hostile, complaining that people were watching him. She was frightened and exhausted and did not know what to do.

I asked them both to come to my office in the afternoon. Considering how upset Mrs. Atkins had been on the phone and how she had described her husband, both seemed remarkably composed when I first met them; first together, then separately, and then, as they preferred, together. Mr. Atkins said he had had a terrible dream about being enveloped in darkness the night before he had put up the notice. Then on the day he had gone to the library, there had been a power blackout which had frightened him even more.

Mrs. Atkins spoke in a tense, somewhat patronizing manner about her husband:

> This has happened before. He gets sensitized. I've had to become his psychiatrist. It's a great burden. I have my own work to do. My scripts are finally being used. But I don't mind. We've been married a long time. I would never leave him.

While she was speaking, Mr. Atkins seemed to bare his teeth and hiss at her through the side of his mouth. He tried to interrupt whatever she was saying, as she did to him whenever he spoke. After listening for some time I suggested that there might be some tension between them, because they both had high-pressured and demanding jobs. Both denied this and added how much they loved each other.

> He added, "It's not disgraceful to be dependent on your wife."
> She replied: "It's not wrong to be the man in the family."

After a few hours, I asked to see them again the next day. They agreed and came on Monday and Tuesday, somewhat refreshed after having had some sleep. They talked a lot about themselves, their relationships, and frustrated hopes for success. Mr. Atkins came from a working-class background, one of two children. He had a younger brother who had died some years before. Significantly, he did not dwell on his brother. His father had ruled the family with an iron hand and only recently had retired. His mother was dead. He was worried about his business. It was not doing well and might go bust. He had had a previous breakdown and had been treated with drugs and ECT.

Mrs. Atkins came from a middle-class background. Her father had been a distinguished engineer. She had hoped that her husband would be as distinguished as her father. They had two teenaged children, a boy and a girl.

The Atkins repeatedly denied any rivalry or conflict of interests. Almost simultaneously they continued to clash with each other.

These two days proved to be the lull before the storm. On the Wednesday morning they practically rushed into my consulting room.

Mr. Atkins was withdrawn, anxious, disheveled, and unshaven. His wife was crying and hysterical.

> "I can't take it anymore. Peter was up all night cuddled up against me, shaking and shouting. He refused to let me sleep or do anything but look after him. He kept talking about the imminence of nuclear war, the coming world catastrophe. You must do something!"

I had previously discussed the Arbours Center with them and said it might be possible for Mr. Atkins to stay there if he wished. I brought this up again and both agreed it was a good idea. He did not want to go to a mental hospital.

I explained that I would have to discuss his proposed stay with the therapists at the Center, but that I thought it would be OK. While I was making arrangements, Mr. Atkins continued to mutter about his crimes against humanity. However, he had visibly calmed down.

The first meeting at the Center included David Rose, the resident therapist, and Alwina Werner, a member of our training program who was assisting at the Center. I was the team leader. Within a couple of days the team grew to include Diana DiVigili, the other resident therapist, and Marge Rose, David's wife.

We quickly realized that our efforts had to be directed to Mrs. Atkins as well as her husband. Not only was she severely shaken, but she did not want to leave him, even though she did not want to stay with him. Mr. Atkins did not want to remain alone and pleaded with his wife to stay with him. Almost in the same breath he agreed to let her go if we would help her too.

We told Mr. Atkins that we would meet with his wife as well as him, but at that moment, she needed a break. Mrs. Atkins promised to return the next morning, while her husband sank into the couch with a sign of relief, while also exclaiming, "There is no time left, Joe. No hope."

The next day Mr. Atkins seemed to fall apart right in front of our eyes. He had not slept and was very agitated. He continuously blamed himself for crimes against humanity. When his wife arrived, he smashed his eyeglasses while shouting about the need to remain nonviolent.

Our first meeting at the Center was monopolized by Mr. Atkins who cajoled and bullied his wife to write down a detailed statement against the dangers of nuclear war, against violence of all kinds, and for the liberation of the human mind, body, and spirit. This activity was to be repeated many times over the ensuing month. Mrs. Atkins took down every word, meekly at first, later with increasing resentment. She was calmer than the day before. However, one could see how worried she was, especially when her husband went on and on about feeling shell-shocked and seeing the Crisis Center like a concentration camp.

Every so often, Mr. Atkins would interrupt his dictation by declaring, "This is the 11th hour of the 11th day of the 11th month! There is no time left!" (This was the 10th of November. The next day was Remembrance Day!)

Then he would go on with his statement. At one point he stopped, looked me straight in the eye and said, "Joe, do you realize how much this hurts? Do you realize what a hell this is?"

I looked straight back at him and replied, "Yes, Peter, I do."

The 11th of November was terribly important for Mr. Atkins. We did not know why. We thought it might have something to do with his father. He talked a lot about him, with fist shaking and teeth clenched, while preparing another statement about nonviolent revolution.

"You know, Peter, you are talking to me about your father, and about nonviolence, in a very angry way. I feel as if I were your father, a father with whom you are very angry."

"No Joe, that can't be." Mr. Atkins was taken aback by what I said. He could not believe he would treat anyone like his father. He denied he had ever been angry with his father.

Later on what I had said seemed to sink in. Mr. Atkins grew silent and reflective. Suddenly he lunged for me, half aggressively and half wanting to make contact. I held him tightly. He quickly relaxed. Tears came to his eyes.

That day we did not meet with Mrs. Atkins. She decided to keep her distance. She was very guilty about doing so. In the evening I received an anxious call from Mr. Atkins. He wanted me to come to the Center immediately so we could go out and post another notice about nuclear war. We talked awhile and he agreed to work on it with me next day.

Saturday was rather difficult. I came to find Mr. Atkins pacing about the living room, naked. He was demanding to call the police and fire department, claiming he was being held prisoner. He relaxed a bit when he saw me, then leapt up and ran for the door. At that moment David Rose was coming downstairs with a blanket for him. David wrapped it around and told him quite firmly that running around the streets naked is improper. Then Mrs. Atkins came and he collapsed into her arms. She got him his clothes and told him to get dressed for the meeting. He did.

The meeting began with Mr. Atkins trying to put together pieces of a previous statement, one that his wife had meticulously written down for him. The night before he had urinated on it and torn it to pieces. After a while attention shifted, from the dirty bits of paper, to his brother, Mike. Although younger, Mike always seemed to be ahead. He got better grades at school and was a war hero.

"I don't know how he did it, Joe. He built up his business much faster than I did. But I never felt any resentment or hostility toward him. In fact, I used to look after him, the times he got depressed and tried to kill himself."

After a break for coffee and biscuits we resumed the meeting. Mr. Atkins talked more about himself, about the difficulties of building up his business in the 1950s and about one particular visit to London with his wife. They had gone to a restaurant for a meal. When they returned to their car, they saw someone had broken in and stolen a briefcase containing the results of two years' work on a new chemical process. There were no duplicates. For the first time, Mr. Atkins began to cry. Then he recalled that on their way up north, someone had followed them on the motorway. It was night. Two people were in the car, a man and a woman. No matter what he did, he could not pull away from them. Mr. Atkins broke into anguished sobs, screaming and kicking his feet. David held him in his arms until he calmed down. It seemed that more than forty years of feelings had finally begun to emerge.

We stopped for lunch. For the rest of the day Mr. Atkins was quiet, lucid and not psychotic.

If Saturday had been the day of catharsis, Sunday was the day of decision, for ourselves as well as for the Atkins. Mr. Atkins had awoken early and gone to church. On his return he wandered into a "blind alley" and had thought of climbing a parapet and jumping off. When Mrs. Atkins came he was reserved and cold. In the meeting he talked about his mother (she had been a religious woman), and about his childhood. He admitted that there were times when he had been mean to his brother. Once he had pushed him off a tree and Mike had gashed his head and bled profusely. He thought he had killed him. However, in recalling this, there were no outbursts, no tears and few feelings. Perhaps these had gone into the therapists. Mrs. Atkins was terrified. She wanted to leave and never come back. The day before Mr. Atkins had buried himself into her arms. She did not want to catch him again. David and Marge were bleary from lack of sleep and Diana felt fragile and battered. I was worried that Mr. Atkins might accidently kill himself just as he was starting to get better (the suicide risk is greatest at this point); but I was especially worried about the others, who seemed at their wits' end.

The therapists needed to be more supportive of each other. We did this by holding a few extended meetings (in contrast to our frequent but briefer exchanges of information) where we concentrated on what we were feeling, in addition to what we were doing. In this way we gained considerable relief from the tensions and antagonisms that had developed over the previous week, because we were able to relate them, and other feelings as well, to what we were holding or containing on behalf of the Atkins. For example, while we were thrashing this out, Mrs. Atkins recalled several incidents from her own childhood which allowed her to appreciate why Mr. Atkins had become so frightening to her. With this realization she felt better and no longer wanted to leave. This process enabled us to renew and enlarge our own emotional space which was in danger of being used up.

Secondly, we decided to be more structured in our work with the Atkins and thereby limit the drain on our resources. We thought that Mr. Atkins could tolerate this because he had made good use of the meeting over the weekend and was somewhat less fragmented in his thoughts and actions. I proposed to see him in analytic therapy once a day at a set time for one hour. Diana agreed to see Mrs. Atkins twice a week, also for one hour, and we all agreed to hold one formal family meeting every Thursday afternoon. We discussed this with the Atkins and they agreed to this plan too.

Thirdly, we decided to review our policy on medication. We had discussed this with Mr. Atkins at the beginning of his stay. He said he did not want any medication (except for an occasional sleeping pill) because he had been heavily tranquilized before and it did not do much good. We concurred because we prefer not to rely on psychotropic drugs at the Center. However, under these circumstances, I said that if Mr. Atkins had not become less agitated and more cooperative within three days, I would recommend a modest amount of phenothiazine. In fact, we did obtain a prescription for Stelazine the next day, but it was never used. Significantly, the resident therapists commented that just because Stelazine was available, they felt much better and able to carry on.[5]

Mr. Atkins slept through his first appointment with me. Later he complained of being blind. Diana said he was keeping his eyes shut. When I came the next day I suggested that he had kept his eyes shut because there were things he still did not want to see about himself. He agreed and casually mentioned that his brother had killed himself some years before on the 11th of November. He quickly added that this date had nothing to do with his current breakdown. I did not contest this denial at the time, but over the ensuing weeks we discussed this anniversary at length. Mr. Atkins began to realize how guilty he felt about his brother's death and how much he wanted to join him in the grave. Moreover these wishes were evoked at any time he became rivalrous and hostile with brother substitutes, such as at times his wife. In fact, it gradually became clear that the crisis, both in Mr. Atkins and in his wife, had been provoked by his wife's increasing success as a writer.[6]

Throughout the next four weeks Mr. Atkins persisted with the therapy, and continued to become stronger emotionally, mentally, and physically. Of course there were ups and downs and brief periods of very disturbed behavior. Generally, however, he moved from a fragmented, disorganized, confused, and regressed state to one that was appropriately depressed and genuinely insightful.

I would like to review one particular session early in the therapy. It demonstrates that residues of psychotic behavior continued to be present during the early weeks of his stay and that they were relieved by the correct interpretation of the transference in the therapy (and also in day-to-day encounters at the Center by the resident therapists).

On the second Saturday at the Center, Mr. Atkins apologized for having raised his voice earlier in the day. He described a dream he had had, about a pyramid of bodies covered with blood. I asked him if they were cadavers. He replied, "No, they weren't." Then he looked away momentarily.

"What occurred to you just then?"

"I was thinking of Andrea. He had a guillotine and was about to chop my head off."[7]

I replied, "I think you fear me in the same way, like an executioner, like Andrea, like your father, like your bad, angry conscience, which threatens you with the direst punishments for any transgression, such as not being perfect." (This was an issue that had previously come to light.)

Mr. Atkins suddenly froze, spat on the floor, looked at me, spat at my glasses, stopped, and cried. He came over and flopped into my arms. I held him for a minute. Then he got up, took my glasses, and slowly tried to wipe them clean.

A few minutes later Mr. Atkins took the glasses into the kitchen. I sat waiting for him to return. When he did, he placed them on a drawing done by another guest, a young girl, which was of a big sun with red marks on and around it.

> The glasses are like the sun, a source of knowledge, insight, understanding, all the things you want from me. You attacked them because you were angry about my being away last night. When I'm away you feel as if I have deprived you of all my knowledge, all the good things you want and need. I think you get angry with me, my glasses, my breasts, just as you used to get angry with your mother, for feeding Mike and not you; and just as you used to get angry with your father, for not giving you more; and nowadays, just as you get angry with Susan, when she spends her time writing and not looking after you.[8]

Mr. Atkins nodded in agreement. He was curiously childlike and did not seem to be able to speak.

"I think what I'm saying is confirmed by the drawing you have brought in with the glasses. The sun also represents my breasts. The red marks represent blood, your teeth marks, your angry biting attacks on me, on mother, on father and on Susan for being away and frustrating and depriving you."

I paused before adding, "When you bite me so, I think you also become frightened that you will destroy the sun, the glasses, my breasts, me, so you try to get rid of your anger by locating it somewhere else, in me. When you do this, I appear to you as an angry, biting mother and father conscience, ready and eager to chop off your head, your vital organs, your source of supply in revenge for your attacks on me."

Mr. Atkins remained seated, deeply attentive.

"You also have a strong wish to clean things up, make things better again. I think you tried to put things right and undo the damage when you tried to wipe the dirt off my glasses. When you can't make things perfectly right again, whether with my glasses, or yourself, you get furious with yourself, and very depressed."

After some further discussion Mr. Atkins got upset. "I'm worried that I won't be able to remember everything we've been talking about."

"I think what I say is like food to you. When you are very hungry, such as now, before the end of the session, you eat up, take in what I say in an angry, greedy manner. Then my words, the food becomes all mangled and destroyed inside you. You can't remember what I have said because you don't want to keep all this chopped up, bitten up, food inside you."

Mr. Atkins sighed and became very still and calm. "Joe, it's like a miracle today. I have some hope at last. I'm beginning to think I may get over this."

It was the end of the session. Before I could go Mr. Atkins recalled that the next day was Sunday.

"Joe, you need a day off."

I thanked him and said I would see him on Monday. He was both being generous and acting upon his fear that if I came every day of the week, he would drain me and there would be nothing left. I didn't mention this at the time. He brought it up of his own accord later on in the week. He was pleased I had waited till he could make his own interpretation.

While Mr. Atkins was progressing, Diana DiVigili was meeting with Mrs. Atkins twice a week, and we all got together for a couple of hours once a week.

Initially Mrs. Atkins found it very hard to talk about herself. She seemed determined to demonstrate her intensive knowledge of her husband's feelings and problems. She seemed to think it was wrong to have concerns of her own. But some gentle questioning revealed that she was desperate to talk to someone. She had no close friends and she could not turn to her husband. She often felt as if she were going crazy. She said that she could never leave her husband, but admitted that she did not want to stay with him, especially when he would infuriate her with his demands. She had her own work to get on with. She had joined a woman's group back north, but it did not help much, because she could never get away from Mr. Atkins. She often had thoughts about him dying in a car crash. Then she could get on with her life. She reckoned that she had ten good years of writing left in her and she wanted to be successful before she was old and could not enjoy life.

Mrs. Atkins was also very frightened of her husband, especially when "he got sensitized" and aggressive. So she humored him and belittled him, in order to keep him "small and docile," a good little boy who would let her get on with her own work in relative peace. This did not always work and she was often depressed.

The family meetings were tense, but very productive. I began them by commenting that the meetings were to help them look at their relationship together. At first Mr. Atkins seemed frightened of his wife. He accused her of not being interested in his manifesto. She denied this. He accused her of not taking him seriously. She denied this too in a high pitched, patronizing tone of voice. I suggested that Mrs. Atkins might find it hard to appreciate how much her husband was changing, and that it might be possible to consider a new partnership, where she did not have to mother him, or be his psychiatrist, and he did not have to be so clinging and demanding. The Atkins seemed surprised that a change was possible, and that they did not have to avoid each other, even when they were talking to each other. Over the years this ritualized avoidance served to dampen the antagonisms between them. What they had not realized was that it also blocked out the large amount of affection they still had for one another. The therapy did not just mobilize their antagonisms, it opened their eyes to this affection as well. By mid December, the Atkins were doing things together for the first time in years, like going shopping, visiting museums, and making love.

Altogether, Mr. Atkins stayed at the Crisis Center for five weeks. As might be expected, it was not easy for him to leave. But he had business to attend to and Mrs. Atkins wanted to get back to the children. I recommended that Mr. Atkins continue in psychotherapy upon his return home. He was willing to do so. Unfortunately there are not many psychotherapists in practice north of Manchester, so this has proven to be a difficulty.

A week after leaving the Center, Mr. Atkins phoned and thanked me for all the help. He was fine, business was good and Susan had landed a big contract. Three months later he wrote to Dave and Marge, again thanking them for all their help and sending best wishes to everyone. Both his business and family life had never been better.

I have often been asked, "How is it possible for someone to go through a deep depression or psychosis so quickly, what do you really do at the Crisis Center?"

The point is that if this experience is a response to a life crisis, then the affected person has already entered a state where his personality, his character, his whole life are rapidly changing. My role is to assist this change, to enable it to occur as fully and profoundly as possible, not to delay or retard it.

Sometimes such changes may occur in a person who is already in psychotherapy or psychoanalysis. This was the case with Danny, a 40-year-old American artist who had moved to London after achieving considerable success in New York. Danny had initially consulted me at a time of great unhappiness. His marriage had broken up and he was uncertain whether to paint, sculpt, or devote himself to teaching. After several years of therapy the dragon of his self-destruction lay quiet and his work took on a colorful new direction. Then his mother died. She had been the dominating figure in a large extended family. Her death evoked relief and grief, seeming unconcern, and a strong attachment to a younger woman who was, "the first with whom I could be openly aggressive and angry." Then she left him and Danny became distraught. For him this loss confirmed that he could never express his feelings, that his destructiveness knew no bounds, that no relationship was safe. He was convinced that the few friends he had left were plotting to kill him and that I was just waiting for the right moment to get rid of him.

"I'm rubbish, nobody wants me, nobody can stand me. I want to go to mental hospital. I want drugs to put me to sleep, forever." However, Danny could still reflect on what was happening to him. Intermittently he thought that he might be better off if he did not go to a hospital but tried to come to grips with his feelings. As he knew about the Crisis Center, he asked if he could go there and still have his regular sessions with me. I agreed.

Danny stayed at the Center for four weeks. The Center became his chrysalis, a place where the most profound changes in his feelings and outlook could take place while he was safe and protected from all outside pressures. He has eloquently recalled his breakdown, the first days at the Center and a long dream which presaged his recovery.

The Breakdown

It didn't happen all at once, rather gradually over several weeks. My depression got worse and I couldn't cope with work, with everyday chores about the house, with even answering the phone. I was drinking very heavily and smoking of lot of pot. In the past this would help, but then it just made everything seem more negative. This culminated in the terrifying week before I went to the Center when I became frightened of everyone around me and didn't want to go out of the house. I couldn't talk to anyone, or even to myself, I found it impossible to make any kind of reasonable explanation of the situation. I finally ended up with a complete sense of fragmentation. Literally I felt fragmented, shattered. I was a victim unable to control things, a fragment myself, whirling around. Since I was still coming to see you, I was frightened that you wouldn't believe me, that you would think it was all a ploy. It took a whole day before I could really admit to myself that I wanted to go to the Crisis Center.

The First Days at the Center

I arrived in the evening. I was very nervous and stayed in my room for the whole of the next day. Then I went downstairs, for breakfast I think. I met Sally and Tom.[9] There was a very cheerful, competent atmosphere. I found it very easy to build a personal relationship with Sally. I suppose I needed a woman, especially a woman with whom I wasn't having a sexual relationship, but who would be there when I felt black and gloomy, someone to talk to. I remember feeling like a derelict black, a Bowery bum, broken and beaten. In the beginning it was so bad I thought I was in hell, then slowly, gradually the gloom began to lift. I found it would help if I could be useful, get involved in doing things like washing up, preparing food, cleaning, things like that. I also decided to do a lot of drawings, to record my dreams, my fantasies. After a couple of days another fellow came, Ritchie I think his name was, a salesman who saw monsters. I took to him right away, and I did a lot of drawings with him. He had never drawn before, but once he got started it was terrific, all sorts of images came up. We did mandalas, together and then with everyone in the house. Otherwise I spent my time going for walks in the park. When I was in the park I would just try to let everything down, immerse myself in my fantasies. Mostly they continued on the theme of degradation, being a degraded figure, and of sad, haunting, gloomy images. Then I had an extraordinary dream, different from anything I had ever dreamed before. In every way it was a turning point.

The Dream

I was looking for my parents who were lost. I went to Paris to find them, but they weren't there. Somebody said they had gone to Spain, so I took a train and went to Spain, to Barcelona. Then I got a little bus up to the Costa Brava. I found myself on top of a cliff that reached all the way down to the sea. I sat staring at the rugged rocks. It was a bleak and wild scene. Suddenly I had the feeling that I wasn't going to find my parents, that the search had reached its end. This was very painful. I decided to return to England.

Upon my return I was back on the Finchley Road [London] walking to see my friends Mike and Molly. They have always stood for my parents. They have a large family, lots of children. I often visit them and they have looked after me. When I arrived they were just on the point of going out. They said, "Come on, let's all go out and have a drink together." Instead of going to our usual pub, we took a different turn and found ourselves in a completely unfamiliar part of London, where I had never been before, almost like countryside.

I discovered a very old pub on a crossroads. It seemed to have been made at different times. Some parts were very old indeed, perhaps the 14th or 15th century, and other parts were garish and modern. I went into the pub. It was composed of numerous bars and small rooms and I made my way into the main room. Immediately I was struck by the fact that the people there didn't seem to belong to this world. They seemed to belong to another world and I had the strong impression that this pub was a gateway to another realm, a gateway to time travel.

The dream continued with Danny meeting 15th century cutthroats and rogues as well as the archangel Michael (a transformation of his friend), who became his guide. Michael led Danny through time and space, to the gate of heaven and to the pit of hell brimful of demonic creatures.[10]

I knew I had the choice of entering the pit or simply closing the door. I felt that I was unable to enter the pit. So I closed the door and as I did so, the nature of this place occurred to me. I realized that it was a zone between the living and the dead, and that the spirits of the dead could visit the living in this place. I also realized that the search for my parents was continuing, and, in fact, that the search was specifically for my mother. Although she was dead, I had been directed to this place in order to meet her.

At that moment a figure appeared dressed in a black cloak which ran down to its feet. It stood at an angle to me with a cowl hiding its face. As soon as I became aware of it, the figure started to walk across a grassy plain that led out of the veranda. I hesitated but Michael instructed me to follow it. Then he said, "I shall be leaving you now."

The figure was like an hallucination. One instant it would be there, then it would seem to vanish. I followed it over gently rolling countryside, no trees, just endlessly rolling grassy plains. The horizon was at least 20 miles distant, yet every single blade of grass was in clear focus, no matter how far away it was. The light was intense and the grass continued to be in clear focus for mile after mile. I followed the figure in a completely timeless way for what could have been hours or days. I felt relaxed and happy, as intended. I was not impatient. After a while I realized that I had been gradually climbing. Although I was on a gently rolling plain, I had been making a slow ascent. Finally I reached the highest place on this whole plain. The horizon now stretched almost infinitely far on all sides. I was on the top of a hill. Near me there was a flat rock on which the figure had lain down, arms outstretched, face upwards, but still hidden by the cowl. It seemed to be beckoning me. I felt that I had to go and lie on the figure face down with my palms touching its palms. It was as if I were about to be crucified.

I went and lay down upon it. As I did I became aware that the figure was my mother. Then this image of my mother began to undergo many kaleidoscopic transformations. Each was familiar and important to me, as if all my relatives, both alive and dead, were flickering through this figure. Finally the figure became solid and substantial. Suddenly I realized that the person I was lying on was you. I had a terrific feeling of relief and support. All my cares and worries seemed to blow away, all my anxieties ceased. I seemed to lose consciousness and then I woke up.

The Recovery

Upon awakening I felt clear and refreshed as well as immensely reassured. I realized that the Crisis Center was truly a secure and comforting place. Within a short time I made plans to visit my home and begin sorting out the mess I had left behind. I became much more active at the Center, helping with the cooking and cleaning and generally taking a keen interest in everything going on. I also resumed my teaching schedule with a degree of enthusiasm I had not experienced for a long while. While my depression and anxiety did not altogether leave me, they returned to normal, that is tolerable levels. I left the Center two weeks later without the feeling of dread which had hung over me for so long. I could look forward to the future.

Danny's transformation followed in the tradition of John Percival (1974), John the Butterfly Man (whom I have previously described),[11] and the many others who have demonstrated a renewed relationship with themselves and others by a dream, vision or reverie. With Danny the passage from psychic fragmentation to emotional reconstruction was made possible by his unconscious acceptance of the help that Sally, Tom and I could give him. He recognized that we could guide him through the rocks and reefs of his hostility and hatred without our being injured or destroyed and without our leaving him as had his mother, wife and girlfriend. He established us as a solid, substantial presence within himself, and, in so doing, reestablished his belief that reality could be benevolent and it was safe to be sane.

Subsequently, Danny has continued the work begun in his therapy and as revealed in the dramatic events at the Crisis Center. He still gets depressed, but not nearly so severely. He still gets anxious, but he is not incapacitated by it. Generally his life has taken a turn for the better.

Over seven and a half years, the Arbours Crisis Center has been able to demonstrate that crisis intervention is a valid and valuable aspect of community care, as well as a viable and cost-effective alternative to hospitalization in many circumstances. Significantly, we have been able to provide intensive, personal, and highly individualized support without relying on medication or other forms of physical restraint. We have also helped to avoid many problems attendant with *cultural closure*—stigmatization and institutionalization as well as the sideeffects of physical treatments. We have found that even the most distressed person can respond to a calm, containing approach. It is evident that people can take advantage of a life crisis when their distress diminishes and they begin to understand what precipitated it.

The most common condition resulting in a stay at the Center has been acute depression. Other states which people have worked through include acute and recurrent psychoses, severe anxiety, anorexia, anti-social behavior and various family and adolescent difficulties.[12] Frequently these events would clearly be traced and were part of a major turning point in the lives of those affected. Two to four people were usually involved in each of these interventions and they came from all walks of life, from laborer to pop star, from housewife to psychologist. The average stay at the Center was two to three weeks, although many guests only came for a few days and some individuals, particularly adolescents, have stayed for several months or more.

Three follow-up studies covering the period January 1973 through February 1980 have shown that the most frequent outcome for people we helped was for them to return home and carry on with their lives. Where this was not feasible, or where further support was needed, guests moved to a long stay Arbours community, to another hostel, or to the home of friends or relatives.

We have not always been successful. Hospitalization was required in eleven cases. Each involved a person who had had a previous history of hospitalization, or who had, as we later discovered, come to the Crisis Center only after having been cajoled into staying by a relative or friend.[13] These individuals were often not ready to look at their inner turmoil and pain at the time they were with us because "it hurts too much," and, "I just want to turn it off." This is a position one has to respect.

However, others, including people who were very disturbed, did choose to confront their difficulties while at the Center:

> "You probably change all the time, but it was quite an experience staying at the Center, and although the actual change is hard to recognize, I felt I benefited from talking about ourselves. I felt relief that there was somewhere or someone who was willing to help when the alternative was hospital." (Young woman who stayed at the Center with her husband and baby, farmers from Scotland.)

> "Arbours helped bring the fester in me to the surface where, for a time, it made a rotten mess. But, once that was done with, the real healing of mind, body and spirit, began. My obsessions and compulsions are leaving me, i.e. picking up stones to see if life's directions could be found under them . . . *The healing is slow, but it's progressive and sure.* (Nurse)

Many guests commented that the very atmosphere of the Center, the house, the people, the nature of the support had a lot to do with their feeling better.

> "At the Crisis Center you are not made to feel inferior, and in my opinion, if the therapists are willing to live, eat and be with you, they are really interested in your well being. I also found the presence of animals very helpful. When I couldn't talk to people, I could talk to the dog, and he was at times much more comforting than anyone could be. It was not a sterile place, but warm and homey." (Student)

> "I enjoyed the freeness of the atmosphere of the house, specifically being able to have honest, open conversations with strangers whether therapists or patients. I appreciated the communal type living, but wished there had been more organization on cleaning jobs. I appreciated being left alone to my own resources when I wanted it so. There was no sense of intrusion there. Also knowing someone was there to talk or comfort me at any hour if I needed, was a comfort in itself. I was treated with kindness, gentle understanding and respect, and at no time did I feel like a

patient. I responded quickly to the relaxed, calm atmosphere and found answers to questions which had kept me on the edge for years." (Housewife)

In contrast, a few guests complained that there was not enough support because "the staff went to meetings" or that not enough attention was made to keeping the house clean. One person thought the Center was too calm:

"You can express sorrow anywhere, [but] I never saw anyone violent or angry to themselves or others. How do you cope with that?"

Another person wasn't sure whether the term meetings were worthwhile:

"Maybe it helps you realize things, and you think for a time, that's the "reason,' but often it's just a way of looking at it and hasn't solved the problems."

Overall, guests spoke very warmly about the Center and saw both their stay itself and what they had achieved in a favorable light. Their views have been summed up in the words of a young married woman who came to the Center at the time when her marriage was breaking up and she was depressed and suicidal. She left in a different frame of mind:

"The Center is an alternative sanctuary from which I was able, in time, to emerge to find my dignity and my nervous system intact and my potential unprejudiced."

FOOTNOTES

1. When *closure* occurs, it has been found that usually the diagnosis has been decided upon by the family long before the doctor is called.
2. Individual and family consultations and stays at the Center are paid privately, or by council (local government) grants, or by various insurance plans. Allowance is made for people who are not covered by local government grants or insurance and may not have sufficient resources to cover their fees. An essential contribution to overheads is provided by

the therapists, all of whom receive minimal remuneration for their work. Without this, we could never have started the project nor kept it in operation. Even so, the Center runs at a loss of $15,000–20,000 per year.

3.   This person may be using another's difficulties to get help for him/herself. Or, he/she may be suffering an "interpersonal crisis," an acute stress reaction brought about by the threatened disintegration of a relative or friend.

4.   On several occasions we have recommended that people stop taking a toxic level of tranquilization as indicated by lethargy, tremor, and other mental and physical side effects. When the medication was stopped, many of the alleged signs and symptoms of their mental illness also ceased.

5.   The relief the resident therapists felt when Stelazine was available confirms my view that psychotropic drugs are as useful to members of a distressed person's social network as they are to the person in distress. At home this includes family and friends. At a hospital this includes staff and probably other patients. In other words, these people feel better when someone other than themselves is sedated. I have discussed this phenomenon at length in my chapter on psychotropic drugs, "The Girl who Wouldn't Stop Singing," in *I Haven't Had to Go Mad Here*.

6.   A breakdown which occurs on the anniversary of an important personal event, such as the death of a relative, has been called *the anniversary reaction*. Mr. Atkins' psychosis is an example of an *anniversary reaction*. Dr. George H. Pollock (1975) has written extensively about this phenomenon.

7.   Mr. Atkins was referring to Andrea Sabbadina, a team leader at the Center and previously a resident therapist. He had come that morning to meet with another guest.

8.   Later on when I reviewed this session I realized that in taking my glasses from me, Mr. Atkins had wanted to turn me into himself; someone who could not see. This was both an expression of his envy toward me and his wish not to be himself, because to be "Peter" was to feel humiliated and full of pain. He preferred that I be "Peter" instead.

9.   Tom Ryan and Sally Berry were the first resident therapists at the Crisis Center. They are now team leaders at the Center and coordinators of an Arbours Community.

10.   The entire dream has been published in *I Haven't Had to Go Mad Here*, op. cit., pp. 148–152.

11.   I have discussed the metamorphosis of John in Chapter 5 "The Butterfly Man," in *I Haven't Had to Go Mad Here*.

12. Diagnostically the psychoses included acute first time schizophrenia, acute recurrent schizophrenia, and acute manic psychoses. The family and adolescent difficulties ranged from various kinds of marital discord to adjustment reactions of adolescence.

13. Residence at the Center is on a voluntary basis. For us to help them, guests must come and stay of their own accord. Naturally there is some degree of conflict in everyone about facing problems, as opposed to dismissing or running away from them. However, once we engage people in what they see is a meaningful discussion of their concerns, this initial reluctance greatly diminishes.

REFERENCES

Berke, J. H. *I haven't had to go mad here*. London: Pelican Books, Penguin Books, Ltd., 1979.

Bion, W. R. *Learning from experience*. New York: Jason Aronson, Inc., 1977.

Perceval, J. I. *Perceval's narrative: A patient's account of his psychosis, 1830–1832*, Gregory Bateson, ed. New York: William Morrow & Co., 1974.

Pollock, G. H. On anniversary suicide and mourning, in Anthony E. J. and Benedek T., eds. *Depression and human existence*. Boston: Little Brown and Co., 1975.

Segal, H. Psychoanalytical approach to the treatment of schizophrenia, in Lester M. H., ed. *Studies of schizophrenia*. Askford, Kent: Headly Books, 1975.

Chapter 3

FOLK HEALING SYSTEMS AS ELEMENTS IN THE COMMUNITY

Support Systems of Psychiatric Patients

Vivian Garrison, Ph.D.

In this chapter the importance of the linkages between formal and informal mental health systems is clearly demonstrated by an intensive single-case study and an overview of the literature. Full consideration is given to the caveats implicit in the multidisciplinary intercultural systems, stressing the necessity of viewing the systems, and their language, in context as complimentary and supplemental rather than alternative. While the similarities between folk psychotherapy and the orthodox Western therapies is explicated, sight is not lost of the fact that there is maladaptive as well as adaptive functioning within any particular cultural context. An emphasis is made that the individual must be assessed by his/her intrapsychic and social functioning in the particular cultural environment.

The work which is based on Vivian Garrison's years of research, data collecting, personal observations and accounts from many such folk healers in Newark's Puerto Rican community, includes a detailed description of a successful network intervention by one such espiritismo, Rosa, who intervenes effectively and skillfully with a Puerto Rican family crisis on a variety of psychological levels. Through this case, the reader becomes familiar with a

very human family whose belief systems allow its members to trust
a ritualistic healing process which succeeds in crisis resolution for
all family members.

In Newark, New Jersey, a long-term goal is to adapt the mental
health care delivery system to the natural patterns of life in the low-
income and high-risk black, hispanic, and white ethnic communities
comprising the catchment area of the College of Medicine and Dentistry of New Jersey, New Jersey Medical School, Community Mental
Health Center (Thomas and Garrison, 1975). As part of this effort, the
Inner City Support Systems Project (ICSS), a five-year coordinated
research, training and experimental clinical service program,[1] has
focused upon the folk healers of these communities as one possible
element in the natural support systems of patients. These "healers"
include rootworkers, prophets, and spiritual advisors in the black
communities (Baer, 1979; Hall and Bourne, 1973; Jordan, 1975;
Snow, 1979), espiritistas and santeros among the Hispanics (Garrison,
1977b; Harwood, 1977; Koss, 1975; Lubchansky et al., 1970; Rogler
and Hollingshead, 1961, 1965), and spiritualists, psychics, astrologers,
reader advisors, and charismatic faith healers in all communities.
Similar beliefs and practices have come to be viewed as "alternative
medical systems" with distinct but culturally valid "concepts of illness"
and frequently efficacious methods of treatment in some international
health programs (Bannerman, 1977), in medical anthropology (Kleinman, 1978; Leslie, 1976; Press, 1980), in transcultural psychiatry (Jilek,
1971; Prince, 1980; Torrey, 1972) and in scattered mental health
programs in the United States (Abad et al., 1974; Bergman, 1973;
Fields, 1976, Koss, 1977, Ruiz, 1976; Scott, 1974; Weidman, 1978,
1979). The President's Mental Health Commission (1978) noted the
importance of traditional cultural health belief systems and indigenous
healing practices in the "New Forms of Support Systems."
In Newark the Inner City Support Systems project is exploring the
role of such practitioners in the naturally occurring support systems of
patients with the ultimate goal:

to develop an optimal relationship between the folk healers and
the orthodox care system which will *maximize the benefits, minimize
the risks*, and *reduce the conflicts for patients* of the coexistence of
alternative independent systems of conceptualization and management of the same or similar conditions.

Perhaps more importantly, however, the alternative healing systems
generated and perpetuated within distinct cultural groups reflect pat-

terns of help-seeking, help-giving, and help-receiving which permeate the culture more generally and are not specific to the folk healing beliefs and practice. For this reason, the folk practices provide a "royal road" to understanding of norms, values, and habitual patterns of behavior within those communities which can be used as models of styles of service delivery and care giving which might be more amenable, acceptable and, therefore more effective, within the particular culture.

This project cannot be reported in detail here, but will instead be illustrated with a case example of one naturally occurring support system in a Puerto Rican community and one healer's intervention in that system. This case, drawn from an earlier project with similar goals[2] demonstrates the importance for clinical care of an understanding of these beliefs and practices as they are found in community context and suggests some of the potential benefits to be derived from the professional mental health care system from linkage with these healers as naturally occurring supports for patients in culturally distinct communities. The ethical, professional, and institutional issues of implementation of such linkages are, however, highly complex (Bibeau, 1979; Osborne, 1969; Singer, 1976) and will not be dealt with here.

The case to be presented was documented entirely in the community setting[3] and none of the people whose lives were profoundly influenced by this intervention are identified psychiatric patients. They ranged in mental status at the time of this episode from free of significant psychiatric disorder to moderately disturbed. It is a particularly "good case" psychotherapeutically and it is not intended to suggest that all folk healers' treatments are equally impressive. The healer involved, however, an *espiritista* (spiritist medium) and *santera* (priest in *Santería*), is fairly representative of practitioners in these two traditions. Nine of fifteen such practitioners studied in Newark were very similar in their basic beliefs about the nature and causes of spiritual illnesses, their treatment techniques, and their skills in application of these.

Espiritismo is a folk-healing system popular throughout the Spanish-speaking New World. Codified by a 19th century French scientist and mystic, who used the pen name Alan Kardec, it posits the coexistence of two interrelated spheres, a "material, visible world" and a "spiritual, invisible world" of spirits of all.

THE SOCIAL NETWORK AND SUPPORT SYSTEMS OF ROBERT MALDONADO AND HIS FAMILY

Robert Maldonado is an attractive, intelligent and artistically gifted young Neorican (New York-born Puerto Rican). He was 16 years old, in his last year of a high school for the especially gifted, working part-time as a checker in a supermarket, and planning to go to college and prepare for a professional career in architecture, when shortly before his Regent's examination he jumped from a second-story window during a fire. He suffered torn tendons in one leg requiring it be put in a cast. Six weeks later, he had still not returned to school and had missed his exams. His family was worried about his apparent apathy; Roberto was concerned because his leg might never be exactly the same. He complained that he was "completely blocked" on the half-finished shelves in his bedroom and all other projects, "not ready to go back to school," and admitted that it was not his leg—"That is just my excuse." Later, he would say he was "like in a recession period—like kind of easing it out, trying to catch up on things, trying to find my own value."

This was the situation that mobilized the Maldonado family network and the intervention of the *espiritista*, Rosa,[4] to be described. This network and the intervention is complex, involving many families, neighbors and friends in multiplex relationships (Figure 3–1).

Background

The Maldonado family consisted of four generations of women and all of their living offspring, residing in five households in close proximity with frequent contact among them and all contributing to the subsistence base of the total family. Roberto's great-grandmother, in her 80s and blind, lived alone in an apartment in Building 1 (Figure 3–1) surrounded and cared for by three of her six children and a number of neighboring families, including the Riveras. Agustina Rivera was the superintendent of Building 1 and she had either friendly or antagonistic relationships with all who lived there, whether relative, in-law or merely tenant. She also had a long-term relationship with Rosa, the president of one of the three nearby *Centros Espiritistas*. Agustina is a self-contained and controlling person and, although she will not admit to ever having had a problem herself, she had been attending Rosa's center episodically over a ten-year period "accompanying" people she considered to have problems that needed spiritual attention. Her husband, Cirilo Rivera, is an alcoholic and it was frequently to enlist some authority to exercise greater control over his behavior that she came to the center. At times she came looking out for (or interfering with, depending upon who was speaking) the welfare of troubled residents of her building or neighborhood—as was the case with Dolores Nieves, a tenant Agustina was taking to Rosa's *centro* at the time Roberto's grandmother became concerned about him. Regardless of whose problem it was that brought Agustina to the *centro*, she was

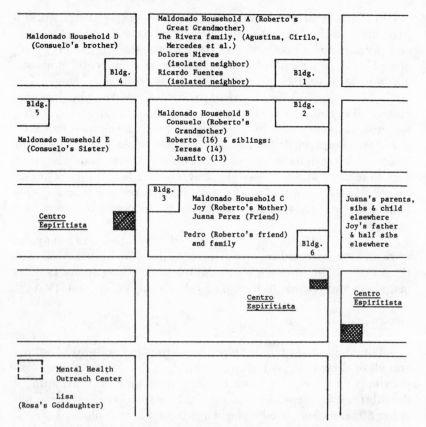

Figure 3–1.   The Maldonado Family and Social Network

always "worked" herself for a *causa de brujería* (work of sorcery) because, as Rosa says: "She is *muy metida* (very nosy), and besides she is super of that building, and she makes many enemies."

Consuelo, Roberto's grandmother, in her 60s, was the fourth of six children, the youngest child of her own father, who died shortly after her birth. Consuelo never married, but in her youth she had a relationship of four years' duration and bore two daughters. The first daughter died when she was less than two years old while Consuelo was pregnant with Joy, Roberto's mother. Shortly after that Consuelo separated from companion and, thereafter, raised her surviving daughter alone. She came to New York in search of a better life when Joy was 12. Joy has periodic contact with her father in Puerto Rico, and with three of nine half-siblings living in New York.

Joy has four children, the first of whom is Roberto, her only child by his father with whom she lived, if at all, less than one year. She was married thereafter for six years and Roberto's three younger siblings—

Teresa (14), Juanito (13), and Manolito (12)—were all born of that marriage. Roberto never knew his father and has no concrete knowledge of him, but reports at different times that he was "a rich man," "an IBM executive," "a man of Italian extraction," perhaps "a mafioso." Four years before this episode (when Roberto was twelve) Joy left the four children with their grandmother, Consuelo, who usually refers to them in casual conversation as "my children."

It is not quite clear what Joy did with her life during the first three years after her official separation from her legal husband, but approximately one year before this episode, when she was 40, she had taken up residence in Building 3 (Figure 3–1) with another woman, Juana Perez, 32. Both Joy and Juana wear short mannish haircuts, jeans, and tailored shirts and are masculine in appearance. Joy is an inspector in a factory where she has worked steadily for 15 years and Juana now works there also on the assembly line. They have a number of women friends from the factory with whom they spend their leisure and recreation time.

Juana Perez grew up with both parents in a stable relationship as the youngest of five siblings, but she reports a lifelong history of "epileptic seizures"[5] and a psychiatric hospitalization at the age of nine. She explains that she would "spend a lot of time outside looking at things, for example, the flowers," and "talking to myself." She says she is still known as "*la loca*" ("the crazy one") in her home town. She came to New York to visit a sister at age 20, worked for four years, had a consensual union of two months and bore a child who was placed almost immediately in a home for the mentally retarded. She then went on welfare, drank a great deal, moved from place to place, living sometimes with relatives and sometimes in furnished rooms, and did not work again until she established this relationship with Joy. She had some periods in which she experienced auditory and visual hallucinations but she never sought psychiatric or spiritist help. Juana visits her parents and two siblings in Puerto Rico once a year and sees three siblings in New York fairly regularly, but they played no part in the episode observed except that she had recently received news that her mother was seriously ill. Juana had also recently been told that she had a cyst on a breast that had to be removed surgically, and she had what she called "a ball in her abdomen" which worried her particularly. Juana was afraid of the operation and had not kept subsequent medical appointments. She describes herself as "nervous," "intranquil," "drinking a lot" and "not caring about life." She was clinically depressed and threatening suicide but she was not delusional or hallucinating.

Roberto at that time had five "best friends," including Pedro, a 19-year-old psychology student who worked nights as a security guard and as a part-time drummer in a Latin band that sometimes performs for *Santería* ceremonies. Roberto says all of his friends are older and that he "can't stand 16-year-olds." Pedro, Roberto's only confidant, however, was having his own problems. His girl friend was pregnant and he "doubted her"—doubted that it was his, "didn't want it" and was "having many fights" with his mother and his girl friend. He reported that his dogs (three seemingly friendly German shepherds) had recently "pulled mother down the stairs and broke her leg."

Like the majority of people who attend Rosa's centro (82%), no one in the Maldonado family and social network, with the possible exception of Agustina, were committed adherents to *Espiritismo* or habitual attenders of *espiritista* sessions. All report their religion as Roman Catholic and, although they all knew something about it, Consuelo and Dolores were the only ones who had had any significant experience with *Espiritismo* prior to this episode. Consuelo tells how approximately five years earlier she visited another nearby *centro* with her elderly mother and sister and the *espiritista* "worked a *causa*" (spiritual cause[6]) "with her"[7] that "would not let me be happy with any man." Consuelo had "dreamed with" this spirit frequently and had even felt his presence and smelled his odor, but, after the "working" in the spiritist center "he withdrew completely" and she had not dreamed of him, felt him, or smelled him since. The medium, however told her that she would still never feel love for any man, because this spirit had cut those *fluidos* (sensations).[8] Consuelo was content with that, and quotes herself as having said: "All I want now is to educate my children." Since that time Consuelo has maintained an altar in her home and burned candles to various saints and performed other ritual acts for the spiritual "cleansing" and maintenance of her home, but she has not returned to the spiritist center.

Consuelo was very impressed with the spiritual work of the president of that *Centro,* but she, like others, is critical of her domineering and frequently rude manner. Therefore, when Consuelo began to get the idea that "someone might be doing something" to her or others in her family, she asked Agustina for "someone good."

This Episode

Consuelo explains:

> There are times when one sees bad things happening in the house, understand, that the luck of one is changing, and one thinks that someone is doing something, true?

The "bad things in the house" that Consuelo was seeing were the problems of her grandchildren, particularly Roberto's accident. His jump from the window was not necessitated by the minor fire in the apartment. Since then, "He is not going out, except to his work, not for anything—not going to school, not going to the movies, not going dancing, nowhere." Teresa was acting *sinverguenza* (shamelessly) and without *respeto* (without deference to her elders). Juanito was not sleeping well. Joy was not contributing the $20.00 a week to the household that Consuelo expected. "Roberto," she said, "does not want to see his mother."

Agustina told Consuelo about Rosa and described to her the "cures" she had performed with other people in Building 1 whom Consuelo also knew. She told how Rosa had recently "cured" her own daughter of venereal disease and "worked" the *"causa"* that affected the couple. (Agustina's daughter was also under medical treatment and she does not mean that Rosa cured the "disease" medically diagnosed, which is considered "material," but the "disease," or "illness," as experienced by the patient (cf. Kleinman, 1978). She told her about her sister-in-law, Mercedes, who had been treated by Rosa two years before when her husband died and "his spirit stayed with her, wanting to take her with him," until Rosa "lifted" his spirit. She also called in Dolores Nieves to tell Consuelo of her very recent experiences at Rosa's *centro*.

Dolores Nieves was a 46-year-old woman who had suffered a series of losses over the past three years. First, her husband left her for another woman, selling their jointly owned grocery store as he did so. Next her arthritis became so severe that she could no longer operate her beauty salon and had to sell it. Finally, her only son moved to a distant state taking with him her grandchildren, whom she had helped to raise. Most recently the last grandchild left to join its parents. Dolores also had diabetes. For the past months she had spent much of her time at home alone with "headaches," "not feeling well," "feeling lonely, crying a great deal, not sleeping well, losing things," and having her "mind blank" for periods. She sometimes felt she was "going crazy." The doctor, she said, attributed it all to her diabetes. Dolores had been attending Rosa's *centro* for two weeks and was feeling better and looked better. She was told that she had both "material" and "spiritual" causes, and had been treated by massages with two types of oils blessed by San Lazaro for her arthritis, but she was also told that she had a "spirit that wanted to see her in a wheelchair, useless, maimed, crippled in hands and legs"—"so crippled that you can't even lift a comb to your own head." She had been told of a number of *causas*, but none of them had yet been "worked" or "lifted."

The following week Consuelo, Agustina, and Dolores went to Rosa's *centro* arriving early so that Consuelo could have a *consulta* (private consultation) before the *reunion* (group session) began. This *consulta* was not observed, but what Rosa customarily does is to seat the person opposite her at a small table under the altar in the Saint's room of her apartment, where there are candles, incense, cigars, perfumed alcohol *(agua florida)*, a crucifix—all things which attract the guiding spirits and repel the *causas*—and a bowl of water *(la fuente)*, in which the medium may see scenes of the person's life, past, present, or future. She lights the candles, incense, and cigar (she does not smoke under other circumstances), and sometimes rubs perfumed alcohol on her own or the client's forehead, temples, and back of the neck, and calls upon her "protecting" and "guiding spirits" for assistance in the work to be done. After reciting the Lord's prayer and sometimes one or more *espiritista* prayers, her body moves back and forth gently or jerks rapidly several times, and she begins to speak about what she is "seeing" or "being told by the spirit guides" about the problems of the client.

The first part of the *consulta* usually consists of a series of positive statements about the problems or symptoms to be simply confirmed or denied by the client, e.g., "You have headaches, don't you?" or "You have much fighting in the home?" Once the presenting complaints are divined in this way, the *consulta* continues with more open-ended questions about the history, e.g., "Have you seen a doctor about that?" or "Is this your first marriage?" Each set of symptoms probed are given a spiritual diagnosis or interpretation, which may be a "material" or a "spiritual" explanation, or both. A "material cause" is any natural explanation recognized by the mediums in the physical, social, psychological or historical circumstances. Referrals are made to doctors, social agencies, and, even psychiatrists for those problems the medium "sees" as "material" or about which she does not "see" a spiritual cause. A "spiritual cause" is an etiological explanation based in the spiritual theory of interactions between the living and the "invisible world" of spirits. The symptoms of "spiritual" etiology may be physical, social, or psychological and they may be acute, episodic, or chronic as indicated by the timing of first and subsequent appearance(s) of the spirits. The reasons given for a spirit's attachment to an individual may be current and/or past interpersonal conflicts *(brujería)*, deaths of loved ones, personal history (e.g., spirits with one's parents when one was young), or family history (e.g., "spirits that come with the family" or that "entangle the family"), unresolved relationships in a past life, or the state of "spiritual development" of the person, or a combination of these.

These interpretations may be given as the questioning progresses or at the conclusion of the *consulta*. In either event, at the conclusion of the *consulta* these interpretations are usually repeated and remedies *(remedios)* prescribed. Remedies may be pragmatic problem-solving "material" advice *(consejos)*, ritual acts of cleansing *(limpieza)* or alleviation *(despojos)*, prescriptions *(recetas)* for herbal baths or teas, prayers, amulets, candles to be burned, or advice to follow a more complex regimen of spiritual treatment, such as "having the spirit worked" *(trabajando la causa)* in a *reunion* or "developing spiritual faculties" *(desarrollo espiritual)*—a lifelong process.

In the *consulta* with Consuelo, Rosa elicited the history of the problems in the Maldonado family much as I have described them above. There was no confirmation of Consuelo's vague suspicions of *brujería* and no spiritual or material *causas* were diagnosed except that Rosa did note that she has "a very big *prueba material*" (material trial/ test)—"having an only daughter lesbian." Rosa empathized with Consuelo about this and her concerns for her grandchildren and offered to visit her to do "a spiritual cleansing of the home" *(una limpieza de la casa)* and to see what she could do for Roberto.

During the *reunion* that evening Dolores was one of the handful of people who are selected for intensive "working of the *causas*." The standard spiritist *reunion*, similar to a psychodrama consists of three distinct parts: *(1)* "preparing the atmosphere" or "developing the union of thoughts," *(2)* "working the *causas*," and *(3) despojos* (ritual "cleansing" or "alleviation" of the bad *fluidos* that may remain from having been in the presence of "the dead" there that evening). During the first part, spiritist prayers and passages from "The Gospels According to Spiritism" by Kardec are read aloud, everyone concentrates on God and the guiding spirits. The mediums, seated around a table covered with a white cloth and bearing the same ritual objects as described on the table for the *consulta*, call upon their spirit guides and enter a trance state with their principal guide *(guía principal)* to prepare their bodies for the work of the evening. During the second phase, individuals are called′ forward to the table one by one and all the mediums focus their attention upon that one person "giving them whatever the spirits give them," similar to the process of the *consulta*, but, unlike a *consulta*, also "working the *causas*," if indicated. "Working the *causas*" designates both this stage of the *reunion*, and the specific actions of "mounting," "interrogating," "educating," and "lifting" the molesting spirits.

This evening, Dolores was given the *Gospels According to Spiritism* to open during the preparation phase. In *Espiritismo* it is believed that the passage to which the book is opened will be particularly relevant for the problems of the person who opens it. This act is also a signal to the mediums that this particular person is to be "worked" that night. Dolores was therefore the first one called to the table. A male medium, Francisco, who is considered especially good at "giving *evidencias*" (visual evidence)[9] began the "working" of Dolores by describing a scene of her life that he was "seeing." It involved a small basket suspended from the ceiling near a door where someone kept things. The other mediums interpreted this *evidencia* as indication of a "service for the dead," or a "work" of *brujería* to coerce the spirit of someone deceased to do what the petitioner wanted it to do. The scene was then elaborated with details of a neat woman getting up on a little chair, without her shoes, to tend the basket, changing the fruits, candies, honey, and other things that the spirit likes. This was interpreted by the mediums to mean that there was "a work of retention." The woman who had done a work to Dolores to take her husband away, it was declared, was also doing a "work of retention" "so that he would never leave her house." This woman was also supposed to be "renewing" periodically the *brujería* that originally separated him from Dolores. She was told she had many *causas espirituales*, from these and other sources (a small shrunken woman dressed in black with a rosary, another "that died of thrombosis, or something like that,"[10]) but this evening only one was "worked." This was a male spirit "that comes into her house at night" and "disturbs her sleep by perturbing her thoughts." The medium described how "Instead of getting in her bed, he puts himself at the bottom of it and makes her feel heavy and like she is falling . . . as if she were sinking in her bed." She confirmed these sensations. The spirit was said to want to cause her damage. "It hides things from her sometimes so she cannot find where she left them," and "it takes her mind away sometimes." This spirit, said to have been with her two or three years, was then manifested in the body of a medium in trance and, after calling the mediums "busybodies," arguing with them awhile about doing what he wanted to—not what they wanted him to, and threatening to leave, he repented and began to confess what he had been doing to Dolores:

> *Causa:*   So many pains and discomforts I have brought you! And I wanted to give you a cerebral attack! But, for anyone who has eyes to see, here are these discomforts. (The spirit is now tapping the hands of the medium over the bowl of water, purportedly disposing of the ills that it has caused Dolores.) Because you were suffering some time from nausea—nauseas that they wanted to destroy your stomach. It is true that you have felt dizzy? Is it true that you felt that you were going to fall?
>
> *Rosa:*   You are the one that has her vacillating from one state to another.
>
> *Causa:*   Remember three years ago, what happened to you, and what a different woman you were then? Let the peace of God be here, because the time is short. Because, peace and justice, I am going to detach myself from your right side. And it is not only to you that I have done damage, but to someone else, and here I

throw away these chains that were to prevent you from obtaining happiness in this life. How sick I feel, because I thought I was a child, because they went to find me in a cemetery recently dead. Because you are going to die slowly. Do you want to take off that hospital gown? Because they wanted that you should have an operation that in the x-rays they would find a spot, an ulcer, *in order that you would not be a woman. Because, what rage, so great, at not being able to succeed!* Let the peace of God be here.

The "spirit" left and Dolores was then cleansed spiritually of the *"fluidos"* that might be left with her after the spirit was gone. She was also given a *receta* for perfumes and baths to continue "cleansing" herself of the *fluidos* of this spirit, which having been with her for so long, would have left some of its effects deeply penetrated in her being and these would have to be alleviated *(despojado)* gradually. If this spirit was not fully repentant (as the mediums suspected), it would return and have to be "worked" again.

During the final stage of the reunion, the mediums, in trance with spirit guides, move among the attendees, cleansing each spiritually with various rituals and answering questions that anyone may put to them. Everyone is very active during this period and there is a great deal of touch. Everyone "cleanses themselves" *(despojarse)* by rapidly rotating the hands about the head, some may be brushed with flowers or fresh greenery, sometimes people are fumigated, "developing mediums" will be encouraged to try to go into trance and may succeed. At the conclusion of the reunion, as at the beginning, people mill around and talk with each other. After the session this particular night Rosa gave Dolores two of her wigs to be washed and set, explaining that, although she might be too slow to work on hair of living people, she could always do the wigs, little by little, at her own pace.

The following day Rosa went to Consuelo's house to do a spiritual cleansing and met Roberto. She did a "work" for him "with the saints," "so that his leg would cure rapidly and well." This means that she called upon and supplicated the saints (in this case *San Lazaro* and the *Orisha,* or African powers of *Santería)* to aid the healing of Roberto's leg. In return he promised that he would come to the *centro* to thank and honor them if his leg was indeed cured quickly and well. He was also told that he had a *"causa de arrastre"* (a spirit that holds him back or acts as a drag upon him) preventing him from getting ahead, and that he was "in spiritual development" and should come to the center to have his *causa* "worked" and to begin his spiritual *desarrollo* (unfolding or development).

In spiritist theory certain people, like Roberto,[11] were born in this lifetime with the "spiritual and material mission" to "develop spiritual faculties" *(facultades)* and learn to help themselves and help others through the use of these faculties. In this way they are believed to "advance" in their "spiritual mission" toward the state of a "pure spirit" that need not be reincarnated again. All beings *(seres)*, a synonym for spirit *(espíritu)* in spiritism, were created gross, ignorant, dominated by material impulses, and it is the mission of every *ser* (being), living or dead, to develop toward greater light and understanding, formality, wisdom, and the replacement of material impulses by refined sentiments. Each person who is "in spiritual development" has a *"cuadro espiritual,"* or group of helping and hindering, or testing spirits with them to assist in this development. The *"cuadro espiritual"* always contains a guardian angel *(angel guardian)*, a principal spirit guide *(guía principal)*, and any number of other spirits that may be attached to the person to assist them with particular tasks or to trouble and put tests *(pruebas)* upon them to encourage their spiritual growth and strength. The spirits in the *cuadro* may also punish *(castigar)* the person for not doing what is expected or they may withdraw *(retirarse)* or turn their backs on someone who does not "develop."

Roberto was told that he had a *cuadro* of *Indios* (American Indians), and also a spirit guide who was a *Congo* (Congolese) in life, that likes fire. It was this *Congo*, Rosa said, that gave Roberto the impulse to go out the window during the fire and try to save the children in the apartment below. Roberto acknowledged that he had thought about those children at the time. Rosa said he was trying to reach the first story window and get in there to see about them, but, unfortunately, he slipped and fell the two stories injuring his leg. But, he was "a hero, not a coward" in what he had done.

Roberto went to the doctor that week and found that his leg had mended well. The cast was removed. And the following week he came to the spiritist center "to pay his respects to the Saints."

That same week Joy also came to the *centro* for a *consulta*. She says in retrospect, "I was angry and tense, in bad humor and with a bad temper, sad, and lacking in enthusiasm *(ánimo)* for anything." She was very concerned about her girlfriend, Juana, who had just made a suicidal attempt by ingesting 18 sleeping pills, about her son, Roberto, who "broke his leg and was not going to school," and about her other children who "were not respecting their grandmother." I did not observe this *consulta* either, but I was sitting in the kitchen of Rosa's apartment when Joy came out of the Saint's room, sat down, and recounted what she had heard in the *consulta* that was just too important and too extraordinary for her to not relate to someone immediately—even a stranger. Rosa had told her that she was supposed to be born a male, but, when her older sister died, while her mother was pregnant with her, her mother had wanted another girl so badly and had prayed so hard for a girl, that her sex had been changed in the womb. Consuelo later said to me "It is true. She should have been a man—she looks like a man. It is true that I wanted a girl so badly that . . ., a misfortune *(desgracia)* for us both."

When I asked Rosa about Consuelo, Joy, and Roberto, she said of Joy, that her problems were entirely "material," that she is homosexual and that is "a misfortune of birth—it is in the blood, in the desire." "These are things that you cannot change—you must help her, give her caring *(hacerle la caridad)*—you cannot disparage her *(despreciarla)*." "The intimate things of one, are intimate," she concluded. "But," she said,

> the boy can be helped. He comes in spiritual development. He "has a *cuadro de Indios*," but he is ashamed *(avergonzado)* and has a complex *(complejo)* because he never knew his father, and he was raised by his grandmother because his mother is a lesbian. This affects him deeply in his intimate life.

I asked what she would try to do for him, and she said:

> "I will insist that he goes to school, and I will consult with him with reference to his complexes regarding his mother."

Upon Roberto's appearance at the *centro* with the news about his leg, Rosa did not immediately proceed with any ritual treatment but, instead, talked with him and hired him to do some repairs in the small apartment building which she owned. (Remember that Roberto was "blocked on all [his] projects.") She also asked him to paint a mural in the *centro* to honor the saints that had cured him, which he did gradually over the following two months. For four weeks he worked at odd hours for Rosa and they talked a great deal about his mother, his grandmother, his protectors, and guides, *Espiritismo* and *Santería*, but he did not attend the *reuniones* in the center, possibly because his grandmother, mother, and Juana were usually there, or, perhaps, because Rosa did not feel the timing was right.[12]

Meanwhile, at the next session in the *centro*, Joy, Consuelo, and Agustina brought Juana to have a *"consulta"* before the *reunion* and to have her *causas* "worked" during the reunion. Dolores also came, bringing Ricardo, a 40-year-old homosexual male neighbor, who was discouraged and worried about his future after the recent loss of his long-term lover and only intimate friend. Rosa was wearing a wig for the first time in the *centro*—one newly set by Dolores. She called everyone's attention to it, extolling Dolores' fine handiwork, suggesting that others have their wigs washed and set by her.

The attention of all focused that evening upon Juana. As the "working of the *causas*" began, Rosa announced:

> Look to this sister here in the red coat (indicating at the same time to Juana to come forward, stand at the table and put her hands over the bowl of water). This child is going to have an operation and soon. The doctors do not find anything materially wrong, but nonetheless when a spiritual cleansing has been done for her, the doctors are going to find what it is that she has, because what she has is internal. . . . She has something spiritual and also something material.

For more than an hour the mediums mounted three *causas* one after another expressing Juana's fears about the operation—that she would die on the operating table, that the doctors would be confused and cut healthy organs, that she was already dead and it was like people were mourning her in life, that she would die of an infection in her blood while in the hospital. . . . All of these fears were expressed as desires of her *causas*, who also wanted "to destroy her," "to see her dead, by any hand, her own, the doctor's, an accident." Each *causa* in turn repented of these wishes and took away his or her effects, begged pardon of Juana, and retired to the spirit world. Alternately the protecting and guiding spirits of the mediums reassured her that she would be well, that God did not want her dead, and that the Archangel San Miguel would protect her. Rosa also prescribed the juice of a tropical palm *(Yagua)* for her to take prior to the operation "so that this tumor will begin to dissolve a little." She was also to say the novena of the Holy Trinity, and was not to worry, that the Holy Trinity would sustain and protect her in the operation.

Juana was not told she was "in development" nor were all of her *causas* worked. She was believed to be a person who could not develop her own protections—she had to have external protection—an amulet *(resguardo)*, or better, necklaces of the Saints of *Santería (collares de Santo)*. She had a *causa* that comes with her since very early in life that cannot be "lifted," but must be "controlled." Rosa, therefore, told her at the end of the session, during the *despojos*, to come to her house to see her privately and to "receive *collares* of the Saints." This is a rite in *Santería*—not part of *Espiritismo*. It is an overnight ceremony in which the initate (godchild) is stripped of old clothing, bathed in herbal substances, cleansed spiritually at the altar of the Saints of *Santería* (the *orisha* or "African powers," e.g., Obatalá, Changó, Yemayá, Ochún, Elegúa. . . .), and the person receives "*collares*" or "*eleki*" (bead necklaces in Spanish and Lucumi, respectively) that have been "fed" with the saints during a major ceremony in *Santería*. These necklaces symbolize the "powers" of the "house" (lineage) of the *madrina* (godmother) who initiates the *ahijado* (godchild). The godchild thereby comes under the protection of the protectors of the *madrina* in a ritual relationship of fictitious kinship that carries the same obligations as that of blood mother and daughter. Juana underwent this ritual later that same week, becoming Rosa's godchild for life.

The following week Consuelo came to the *centro* with her granddaughter Teresa, who was not worked by the mediums. Dolores and Ricardo also came, but attention that evening was focused on others. During all of these weeks Rosa, Consuelo, Agustina, and Dolores had spent a considerable amount of time together in each other's homes. During these visits, in casual contacts, Rosa had counselled Roberto's younger siblings about their relationships to mother and grandmother. Rosa also took Dolores with her to parties and dances and on errands of mercy—involving Dolores in her own active life. Meanwhile, Roberto's mural—an iridescent rendition of Christ on the cross—progressed on the wall of the *centro* and all watched it.

Finally the painter himself appeared in the *centro*. Roberto was introduced to the group as the young man who was painting the mural and there was much expression of appreciation. Rosa explained:

> He has a protection that gives him so much, but since he doesn't give him what he wants, he punishes him. And he has a spirit that wants to see him crippled, a useless young man. . . . Paralytic. If not completely paralytic, paralytic for moments. In important moments he gets paralyzed.

During the "working of the *causas*" Roberto was called to the table and "worked" for "a spirit that wants him to have accidents, that gives him bad humor and rage, and makes him seek fights," and also "a protector that needs light." Rosa, not in trance, but speaking "what the spirits gave her" spoke to him in part as follows:

Rosa:	Do you sometimes have something in your mind that you cannot realize?
Roberto:	I don't understand.
Rosa:	Do you have something in your mind that you can't do?
Roberto:	Sometimes, sometimes.
Rosa:	Some days you feel very inferior.
Roberto:	Oh yes.
Rosa:	Inside yourself, you don't say it to anybody, you feel

inferior. You feel like an internal suffering inside. You feel that you are the worst, you are the worst of anybody.

You are not the worst of anybody. You have all that one can have, although poor, you have something great. But this spirit gives you punishment and punishment until you arrive at where you have to arrive. You haven't passed anything yet of what this spirit wants, still you are going to undergo many tests. You sometimes have your head like this big [gesture of the hands], like it is going to explode? And you have so many, so many things that you cannot realize. And sometimes you have a little happiness like this, then you have even greater suffering, is it true or is it a lie?

Roberto: It is true.

Rosa: Do you have days that you cry inside yourself? And you cried, true, alone.

Roberto: Yes.

Then a spirit guide of the medium came, greeting the table, as the "*protecciones*" do, and talked, again in part, like this:

Spirit: Is it true that you say "Why has God cast me into the world to be so poor?"

Roberto: Yes.

Spirit: "In a family that is so poor that what I want I cannot have." Answer me.

Roberto: It's true.

Spirit: Why is my mother my mother, and why have I been born of my father? What is my father? Who is my father and who are his brothers, and who is my mother, and who are my family? That is what you ask inside yourself, why? Why doesn't my mother help me, and why doesn't my father help me, and why do I have to be attached to this poor old lady.

Then another spirit, "a spirit of shock and trial" came into the medium laughing, cursing, refusing to greet the table, and explaining that he had come dragging chains. This spirit spoke, in part, as follows:

Spirit: So much that I put in your mind, in your mind, in your mind. For what? For what if all is lost? Is it true? Then

for this I push you, I make you hit yourself, I make you
fall, I make you break your leg, put you in the game of.
. ., so that they break you. True that you aspire to a
hard game? [This is a reference to his street life and his
ambitions to be an undercover policeman if he cannot
be an architect.]

Roberto: Yes.

Spirit: Ha, ha, ha, (laughing), you, that you cannot. . . .

The spirit talked of Roberto's ambivalence about leaving home and
having an independent life, and his recognition that his only future
was in schooling and how he acted this out by "first going forward" to
school, and then "backward" "into the games." The spirit ended:

Spirit: They tell me that you might pardon me for all the
             damage that I have done to you.

Roberto: You are pardoned.

Spirit: That you help me for the damage that I did to you.
             That I did not let you be happy, I didn't let you be
             tranquil, your ambition and ambition and all that your
             ambition breaks in your hands. But they tell me that
             now it is enough that you are punished, that I should
             leave you in peace and let you be tranquil, that I should
             go with those that are here at my right, that are going
             to take me to a school where my spirit can see a little
             light and progress because at your side what I am
             doing is defeating myself (hundiendome) more each
             time. And some day I will return, because listen, I will
             return to aid you, because I am coming with you as a
             test (en pruebas) and when you have given me what it is I
             ask of you, we will be all right. [The implication is that
             this spirit will become a protection and guide when it
             has received "light" and Roberto learns to cooperate
             with it.]

Roberto: And what is it that you want?

Spirit: Your mind. To work for you. When are you going to
             put yourself to work [spiritual work], answer me? I
             come with knowledge of causa and I know what I am
             doing. But they tell me that they are going to take me
             where my spirit is going to see light, going to see the
             light that I have not seen. . . .

Roberto did not come to the reunion the following week, nor did anyone else in the Maldonado family and social network. Roberto did, however finish his mural and the week after that he came to the *centro* bringing his friend Pedro, for help with his problems, but also because Roberto was proud of his mural and wanted his friend to see it. Pedro was told that he was "in spiritual development" and that he has a blind Congo protector that likes and helps him with the drums. He was not "worked."

Five weeks later Roberto returned to the *centro* just to tell us all that he had returned to school, had made arrangements to make up his exams, and that everything was fine. But exactly one month after that (and six months after his accident to his leg) he reappeared in the *centro*. This time he had a broken arm in a cast which he sustained in an altercation on the street. Rosa said:

> When you fell and broke your leg, I told you that you have a spirit
> that wants to see you always in an accident, do you remember? And
> now, another accident, and not so much time has passed?

Roberto answered:

> "In truth it was not an accident. I look for it."

The "spirits with" Roberto were worked in much the same way as before, with his *causa de arrastre* that holds him back and his "protector that needs light" expressing his self-contempt, self-doubts, identity confusion and anger, his sometimes grandiose and sometimes antisocial illusions, and his frustrations about achieving his realistic ambitions and potential. This time Roberto did not let the broken arm keep him out of school or interfere in any other way with the rest of his life.

Follow-up

In follow-up interviews, approximately one month after each person had stopped attending the sessions, all parties reported relief of the symptoms and conditions of which they had complained and expressed gratitude to Rosa for her assistance. Consuelo felt that her house was "clean," and that the grandchildren were doing fine. There was a very obvious relief of tensions between Consuelo and Joy. Through the spiritual interpretation of a "sexual transformation in the womb," mother and daughter had come to share each other's guilt and shame about the daughter's lesbianism, and they spoke of each other with affection and sympathy. Juana reported that she felt like a "new person." She had returned to the doctor and the cyst had been re-

moved from her breast. Abdominal surgery had not appeared necessary. Dolores continued to be depressed but much less than before and
she was leading a more active life. She and Ricardo had developed a
reciprocal supportive relationship, cooking for each other and spending time in each other's apartments, talking. Rosa had learned in her
more intimate conversations with Dolores, that her exhusband was
actually spending one or two nights a week with her but most of the
time with his new wife. Rosa's opinion was that "as long as Dolores
chooses to share the love of a man," there was little more that she could
do except "give her caring" (hacerle la caridad) whenever she came
asking, "but," Rosa said, "I am not going to go looking for her in her
house." Ricardo was reassured because the mediums "did not tell me
anything," which means in the spiritist belief system that he must not
have anything "spirtual." He thought that the spiritist centro was "a very
good place to go to be with people that would care about what you are
feeling and help alleviate your loneliness," but he did not avail himself
of this opportunity.

Roberto, after his spiritual "working" but before his broken arm,
spoke about his "protections" with some pride, expressed approval of
the work of the mediums with him and others, was skeptical about the
existence of spirits, although he had great intellectual curiosity about
what are called "spirits" and what spiritists do. He was more interested
in Santería—the "more powerful practice." Both he and Pedro were
interested in my research and like parapsychologists, they kept asking:
"What evidence do you find for the truth of the powers claimed?"
Roberto felt that he would like "to make saints" (be initiated fully into
Santería) one day if he had the money. (This initiation cost approximately $3,500 at that time.)

Pedro, on the other hand, had received "collares," the first initiation into this religion, from another santera since his visit to Rosa but he
had no intention of making the full series of initiations. His account of
what occurred in the centro the night he was there went beyond what
was actually observed to have happened. He elaborated the detail,
probably making a composite of all of his prior experience with Espiritismo and some of his own fantasies. He told us, not only of a blind
Congo protection, that he said "everyone has told me about," but also
about a life in a previous incarnation in which he was "a prince," and
"there was a princess who vowed that [he] would never be happy in
another life." He explained that he "had almost been engaged three
times, but they all left for silly reasons or no reason at all." He attributed this to that spirit of the princess. He feels the influence of that
spirit in his life, for example, when he feels attracted to a woman one
minute and the next feels nothing for her, and in the way he tires of the
women he knows. At the time of this follow-up interview, however, he

was not particularly interested in getting that spirit out of his life or changing his behavior. Rosa would say of him "If he doesn't put his part, I can do nothing."

I followed this family and social network for two years after Roberto's last appearance in the *centro*. During that time there were no further crises, and none of the principals returned to the *centro*, although they kept in touch with Rosa. Agustina, of course, found others in her family, building, and neighborhood who needed "spiritual" help, but she found another medium and another *centro* to go to because she found the research going on in Rosa's *centro* intrusive, which, of course, it was. Roberto, when last seen, two years after his broken arm, was living alone in a small apartment, far enough away from his family that he was not involved in the same neighborhood network, but close enough that he could visit frequently, as he did. He had not had another accident or gotten into trouble on the street again. He was still working in a supermarket and had been promoted to assistant manager. He was continuing his studies part-time in the community college and was still interested in architecture, but was considering other occupations in graphic arts, and had developed other interests. He had a girlfriend about whom he was serious, but he did not want to marry because of his studies. He was grateful to the spiritists and approving of them, but does "not believe," and was no longer interested in pursuing either *Espiritismo* or *Santería*. But, should Roberto suffer another accident, or another "period of recession," Rosa, or "anyone who knows," as Rosa says, will be available "to do him charity" *(hacerle la caridad)* again.

In my view of this case, Rosa's interventions, despite very different guiding theory and rationale of treatment, compare favorably with the goals, techniques, and outcome of professional psychotherapies offered the same people. At the individual level, Rosa's practices could be equated with crisis intervention in which any techniques, including environmental manipulation may be utilized to alleviate the immediate distress and restore the patient to the normal level of functioning. But, the individual treatments provided by Rosa frequently went beyond the alleviation of the immediate crisis and involved techniques more analogous in professional practice to: *(1)* brief psychotherapy, in which the goal is to bring about some awareness of the internal conflicts and improve the person's coping in a future situation (e.g., "working the causes" as in the cases of Roberto and Dolores); *(2)* long-term supportive psychotherapy (e.g., the godmother-goddaughter relationship established with Juana[13]), or, not represented in this case, people with problems of "spiritual development" who are not expected to ever become "fully-develped mediums" and; *(3)* long-term uncovering psychotherapy (e.g., the processes of "developing spiritual faculties," which is described in detail elsewhere (Garrison, 1977a; Koss, 1975, 1977). Rosa also uses techniques reminiscent of resocialization and rehabilitation therapies—the parties, the wigs, and the mural in the cases of Dolores and Roberto.

Beyond all of these individual treatments, however, Rosa intervened very effectively in the Maldonado family system. By reinterpreting and rationalizing Joy's homosexuality in such a way as to make it more socially and culturally acceptable, she relieved tensions between the grandmother and mother, and relieved the grandchildren from some of the pressures they were feeling and acting out. She also freed Joy from the acute sense of guilt regarding her failures of motherhood provoked by her children's problems, which also prevented her from being as fully supportive of her friend Juana in her crisis as she might ordinarily have been. Thus their relationship was improved, relieving some of the stresses for Juana. By offering Juana the continuing support of a *madrina* for a goddaughter, Rosa also freed Joy of some of Juana's dependency upon her. Rosa's intervention with Roberto's three younger siblings may have constituted an effective primary or secondary prevention, precluding later difficulties that they might have experienced.

At the network level, Rosa's interventions, with the assistance of Agustina as a gatekeeper, served to mobilize the natually occurring social networks of the neighborhood in support of isolates, such as Dolores and Ricardo, and to bring consensus to bear on behavioral problems like that of Cirilo's alcohol abuse. Such linkages in a network of people that may be active or dormant at any single time, that do not form a group with self-conscious identity or formal membership, but can be mobilized at any time of need or common interests are sometimes called "quasi-groups" and "action sets" (Mayer, 1966). The social network of Agustina is such a quasi-group and action set for individuals in times of crisis. Rosa has as many such quasi-groups and action sets as she has satisfied clients. The linkages, although dormant (as with the godmother–goddaughter relationship between Rosa and Juana) nonetheless exist and may be remembered and reactivated at any time on one's own or another's behalf. Nearly half (49%) of 180 clients studied in Rosa's *centro* had been there before and many were returning after a considerable lapse in time. In the interim there is no formal group membership, sustained relationship, or singular common interest to provide evidence of this linkage for social network/support system researchers or therapists who might wish to identify them.

Rosa also has many informal linkages to the formal mental health services. She not only makes referrals or takes clients to clinics or hospitals when she sees the need, but she also has a "goddaughter in the religion" who is a community mental health worker. This god-daughter, Lisa, worked for several years in a mental health outreach service very close to Rosa's *centro* and during that time Rosa made many referrals of clients to Lisa for help with problems she considered "material," and Lisa made referrals to Rosa of clients she considered to have "spiritual" problems.[14] Rosa's help is frequently sought by families of hospitalized patients and she sometimes goes to mental hospitals to see and treat patients there, or patients are taken on passes to be treated by her. She has also been observed to arrange for the discharge of hospitalized patients to her care. Sometimes she instructs people with serious psychiatric disorders and little family support, as she did with Juana, to report her as "mother" and "next of kin" if they should happen to become hospitalized.

Espiritismo in the Puerto Rican community is a folk psychology, as well as a folk psychotherapy, a mutual aid association, a network therapy, and a true "community mental health service" in that the healer's interventions are in the living systems of the open community. One could also say that it constitutes part of the community mental health care system, through all the informal linkages, whether or not these are recognized and acknowledged by the orthodox services.

ESPIRITISMO IN THE CLINICAL CONTEXT

When these practices are viewed in community context, the question usually raised is: Do they represent an adequate alternative to professional care? In the clinical setting, however, that question is almost irrelevant—if the folk system had provided an adequate alternative, the person would probably not have become a psychiatric patient. Furthermore, the treatment populations, and, therefore, the appropriate treatments, are not comparable. Spiritist clients as a group are less severely emotionally disturbed and much less seriously impaired in function than psychiatric patients (Garrison, 1977b), although there is a minority of those who are severely disturbed in the spiritist client population as well. Among psychiatric patients, however, *Espiritismo* and *espiritistas* frequently constitute significant elements in the patient's support system[15] even though that system has not been fully effective in relieving the conditions which bring the patient to the clinic.

In the clinical setting the question for patients involved in such healing systems is not whether they represent an adequate alternative to professional mental health care, but whether or not the professional system can provide *more effective* treatment. Can the modern American-trained psychotherapist establish rapport, relate effectively, and establish shared goals for therapy with a patient who has such a different self and world view? If so, is the professional alternative to be offered so superior as to justify alienation of the patient from the folk system, or can it be provided so as to supplement or complement, and not compete with, the care and support received by the patient in the community context?

The first question raised in the clinic when a patient talks of *brujería*, spirits, or *espiritistas* is: Are these beliefs culturally shared, therefore, "normal" in the culture, or are they idiosyncratic, "abnormal" and, therefore, "delusional." Since *espiritismo* as a folk psychology provides explanations of both "normal" and "abnormal" experiences, these beliefs can also be "culturally normal" interpretations and explanations of conditions viewed as "abnormal" by both *espiritistas* and psychiatrists. The questions should therefore be "are these culturally shared explanations of the problems of which the patient complains or are they psychopathological distortions of those beliefs?" And, "Do they reflect maladaptive defenses of the patient or do they serve the patient's more adaptive coping in the context of the patient's habitual level of functioning?"

I ask the reader to imagine what might happen if any of the characters in this drama were to suffer another similar crisis of similar kind and this time go, instead of to the *espiritista,* to the mental health clinic. What would happen? How would they present their problems? How would they be assessed and treated? Would they suppress their self-understandings derived from *Espiritismo* and speak only of the "material" that they consider of interest to "the doctor"? Or would they try to explain their "spiritual causes" to the psychotherapist? In the first instance—a common occurrence in the clinic—would they be judged as "lacking insight," "somaticizing," or "denying," because they do not communicate their thoughts, feelings, and behaviors of concern (which are for them "spiritual") in language meaningful to the therapists? In the second instance, if they did try to communicate their self-understanding in spiritist concepts, how would these be understood and assessed out of context? Would Roberto, for example, be assessed as having "delusions of persecution" if he talked about his "spiritual causes," or "delusions of grandeur" if he spoke of his "spirit guides"? Or might these be judged as self-understanding, therefore "insight," within a very different system of conceptualizing psychodynamics?

What if Agustina, Consuelo, Dolores, or Juana tried to tell a psychotherapist about their "spirits" from "*brujería*"? Would these be considered "paranoid delusions"? Or might they be considered culturally shared interpretations of difficulties which actually permitted the uncovering and expression of previously denied feelings associated with disturbances of interpersonal relations (Agustina), family con-

cerns (Consuelo), the anger underlying depression (Dolores), or morbid fears (Juana).

What if the medium Rosa came to the attention of a psychiatric
clinic? Would she be assessed as having "visual and auditory hallucinations" because she "sees" and "hears" things that others cannot see? Or,
might these be recognized as cultural attribution to supernatural
beings of what are actually highly developed human capacities, ego-
functions, of perception and intuition? What about her trance states,
which she passes in and out of at will and only in the context of her
healing role? Or might this be considered carefully controlled "regression in the service of the ego" (or client's egos)?

Such gross errors of clinical assessment of patients presenting
these beliefs do not occur frequently in the clinical setting because
other aspects of the presenting picture usually lead the therapist to
more accurate judgments in spite of this confusion about content of
thought and perpetual experiences. What does happen in the clinical
setting, however, is that the self-understanding, coping strengths, and
resources for support of the patient are frequently underestimated,
while the degree of psychopathology is overestimated. This occurs
particularly when a therapist fails to recognize implicit connections
between the complaints about "spirits" and thoughts, feelings and
behaviors to which they allude. The "culturally normal" meanings of
these beliefs are as folk concepts referring explicitly or implicitly to
thoughts, feelings and behaviors which are also of concern to the
therapist, i.e., the symptoms probed by the mediums leading to the
spiritist interpretation and the thoughts and feelings expressed by the
"spirits" when manifested by the mediums.

In order to be able to understand the symptomatic or supportive
significance of these beliefs and practices as reported by patients, the
therapist must ask the patient what effects these "spirits" have in the
patient's life and determine whether or not the patient in fact makes
these connections understood in the culture. If these connections are
made, the spiritist interpretation may sometimes appear "insightful"
or at least "supportive" of improved "coping." If these connections are
not made, the spiritist interpretations are more likely to be mere
cultural coloration of symptoms. Patients who are psychotic, delusional
or hallucinating sometimes present such explanations of their problems or report that they are mediums. In these cases, the beliefs in
spirits and in mediumship faculties *are associated with* psychosis, but, in
the community context, as we have seen, these are usually interpretations and explanations of symptoms of much less serious disorder.
There are also, however, in the community context, spirit explanations
of very serious disorders that are difficult or impossible to cure (e.g.,
"spirits" that come from before birth or very early in life or spirits from

"old works of *brujería—brujerías* that have not "worn out" or been "cured" in a reasonable length of time). Such beliefs even when presented by psychotic patients may reflect "insight," rather than "delusion," insofar as the patient recognizes the presence of a morbid condition and has labeled it in a culturally appropriate way. In the clinical picture these beliefs may represent anything—from "insight" to "delusion," and, frequently, they are just part of the patient's history, social milieu, or past coping, and not signs or symptoms at all. They must be assessed in each individual case like any other content of thought for the significance they have in the psychological and social dynamics of the patient's life.

This assessment, although not always easy, can be made by a clinician without extensive detailed knowledge of *Espiritismo*. By first discovering the place of these beliefs and practices in the shared understandings of the social network and support system of the patient and, then, examining the role they play in the patient's intrapsychic and interpersonal functioning, these beliefs can be assessed as the influence of just another interpersonal school of psychology and psychotherapy. In order to do this, however, it is important to discriminate among the many levels of communication involved in *Espiritismo* and to distinguish the mediums' understandings from uses of those communications by the patient.

In most therapies, medical or folk, there are three different social arenas, or sectors, in which illness is perceived and reacted to differently: the "professional," "the folk," and "the popular" (Kleinman, 1978). Following Kleinman, but reformulating his concepts somewhat for present purposes, I would point to the differences in understandings of *(1)* "adepts" (professional psychotherapists or "fully developed mediums"), *(2)* the "laity" (patients, clients, or partially trained students in either the professional or folk systems), and *(3)* the "public" (those who have no adept knowledge and little client/patient experience with the system, either folk or professional, but have ideas about it.)

Rosa, as adept, speaks as one who sees, understands, explains, and treats the problems her clients present in the theory, concepts of causality, and treatment modalities of *Espiritismo*. She talks to clients on at least three levels (invoking or not invoking the appropriate "spirit") as she perceives will best influence them: *(1)* as herself—one who is "humble" *(humilde)*, a highly valued trait, professing no particular knowledge unless "they give it" to her; *(2)* as a medium in trance with an "enlightened," wise, and superior "spirit guide," in which case she is directive and moralistic; and *(3)* as a medium in trance with the *causa* (the base material impulses of the unenlightened ignorant and misguided spirits that molest one), in which state she may cry, scream, whimper, curse, roll on the floor, shout imprecations, make demands, or do anything else that a "low-grade, poorly-developed spirit" might do. For her, Spiritism is "a science as well as a religion" and the invisible world of the spirits is governed by natural laws and the divine will. The existence of the spirits is demonstrated by the empirical evidence of the effects that they produce. For her, "spirits" are abstract concepts in which she firmly believes because of the "evidence" she sees; not as a commitment of faith. Professional psychotherapists can talk with her about cases and, as long as their respective theories are grounded in the facts of the case, they will understand each other as well as two professional therapists from different schools of psychotherapy, although mutual understanding of the respective constructs from the two different systems is very difficult and fraught with misconceptions (cf. Abad and Boyce, 1979; Lubchansky, et al. 1970).

The clients, on the other hand, perceive and interpret what Rosa—as herself, or as spirit—says with more or less distortion depending upon their capacities to relate to what the medium is able to intuit. Clients may use these communications for greater self-understanding, for improved coping, or for reinforcement of maladaptive defenses as when a client instead of having the *causa* "educated" and "lifted," uses these interpretations as rationalization for further thoughts, feelings and behaviors of the kind that gave evidence for the existence of that spirit. Sometimes they may be relatively uninfluenced by even the most complex "working." In the psychiatric clinic setting, these beliefs frequently reflect the patient's psychopathology as much as or more than the folk belief system and practice as found in the community. Many misunderstandings of *Espiritismo* have resulted from and been reinforced by experience of clinicians working exclusively with psychiatric patients in whom these beliefs are frequently distorted. For patients, these beliefs are frequently concrete and absolute, not subject to empirical questioning. Patients also frequently believe exclusively in *brujería* as a cause of their illness, but have little or no belief in *Espiritismo* as a means of alleviation. They frequently have little knowldege of the complex self and world view that guides the practices in the spirit *centro*. Nonetheless they may be supported by participation and acceptance in a spiritist group.

The public, or popular, view of these practices is another thing again. The lay public and the satisfied or unsatisfied prior client, the "curiosity seeker," and the public media, represent these practices as mysterious and supernatural. They will talk about how the mediums "told" them things no one could know—giving names, dates, etc., how "miraculously" they were "cured" and how awesome it all is. Attitudes toward it run the gamut from total opposition to it as a sin (the official Roman Catholic position; see the Baltimore Catechism, McGuire,

1962), or "the work of the Devil" (the Pentecostal position), or "ignorant superstitions of the lower class" (a middle class attitude, although
there are also many middle class adherents (Koss, 1977), through
tolerance or occasional use, to full commitment. Clients' or patients'
reports of these experiences and those of family members are also apt
to be reconstructed in the mystical idiom of the popular sector. These
popular level understandings, when accepting, are also supportive of
patients, particularly when shared in the patient's family, as they serve
to shield the patients from the stigma of "mental illness" within their
own community.

In the Inner City Support Systems Project in Newark, the clinical
and supportive significance of these beliefs and practices as reported
by patients are being assessed on an individual basis for each patient
and each healer. The project originally identified 86 practitioners of
various forms of "spiritual" or "occult" healing and counseling in the
Newark communities, including 23 Puerto Rican, Cuban, and Domini-
can *espiritistas* and or *santero(a)s*. Each of these practitioners was contacted, and selected representatives of each tradition, including 15 of
the Hispanic healers, were studied in depth. These depth studies
included not only ethnographic observations and interviews, but also
an ego functions assessment (Bellak et al., 1973) and a clinical skills
assessment done by a psychiatrist.[16] Thereafter, the ethnographic field
workers, familiar with the belief systems in the communities and with
the individual practitioners of the Newark area, entered the Psychiatric
Reception Center and Crisis Clinic as "culture specialists" to work as
special members of the treatment team with teaching, research, and
service functions. As teachers, they fed back to clinical staff the results
of the research in the community and provided guidelines for understanding of these subcultural practices. As researchers, they did extensive "community support systems assessments" (Garrison and Podell,
1979) of consecutive samples of admissions and "intensive case studies"
of patients whose support systems included folk beliefs and/or practices. In the clinical function, the culture specialists collaborated with
the treatment team in implementing and documenting experimental
treatment strategies with patients who were either deeply convinced of
folk beliefs or currently involved with healers. In these experiments
the patient's supports within the community were taken as the base
upon which to build a more effective psychotherapeutic intervention.
These strategies sometimes included accompanying the patient to the
healer to document the reciprocal interactions of the two systems
impacting on the same patient in "natural experiments." Other times
they included bringing the healer to the clinic to consult to the clinic
staff or to the clinic staff and patient, or sometimes, taking the patient
to visit a healer for consultation. More frequently, however, these

experiments did not involve the healer in direct liaison, but instead involved working with the patient within his or her own subcultural constructions of the influences in their lives.

The detailed review here of a single case from one folk healing tradition, and the complexities of assessing the clinical and supportive significance of these beliefs and practices in patients' lives illustrates both the potential and the difficulties of the task we have undertaken. The complexities are compounded manyfold when one also considers the variety of distinct traditions of folk and nonorthodox healing that exist in the contemporary United States, the diversity among healers within each of these traditions, and the issues of legitimation, licensure, compensation and cooptation. From our experience, we have, therefore, concluded that, in the present state of knowledge, any programmatic efforts involving blanket policies with respect to such practitioners in American communities would be premature. But the alternative, to continue to ignore the existence of these practitioners and to treat such beliefs of patients as nonexistent, as part of the illness, or as "religious beliefs" unrelated to mental health is hardly preferable. Our compromise—until these issues can be resolved—is to approach the problem exclusively in the context of standard clinical decision making with each healer's intervention and each patient's use of that intervention being judged on an individual basis.

This conservative approach, in which we merely acknowledge beliefs and practices in the lives of patients and attempt to work within them, may, however, bring about a change in the interrelationships between the folk and the professional systems tantamount to establishing a policy-directed program. Consider, for example, the potential of an informal clinical liaison with Rosa. If she were contacted as a "significant other" in one patient's support system and a consultative and collaborative relationship was established with her around one case, that might institutionalize all of the existing informal linkages, providing the mental health care system with:

1. Access to adept consultation about the "normality" or "abnormality" of the spiritist beliefs of other patients and, therefore the information needed to avoid or reduce the conflicts for patients of being "caught between two worlds" of apparently irreconcilable alternative explanations and prescriptions for management of the same problem.

2. Outreach to the many quasi-groups and action sets which surround her for earlier intervention in cases of persons severely disturbed who would in the natural course of events probably become psychiatric patients only after *espiritista* interventions had failed.

3. The potential for input of professional expertise in the *espir-*

itista's treatment of cases that she felt she could not manage
or that the professional perceived as mismanaged, thus reducing risk of detrimental folk treatment.

4. Opportunity to monitor the health and well-being within the
community context of any identified patient that happens to
also be her client, or to develop collaborative strategies in
which the patient receives support and treatment of "the
spiritual" in the community context while receiving che-
motherapy or other professional treatment of "the material"
simultaneously, thus maximizing the benefits of the supportive services of the *espiritistas* and reducing the costs of these in
the clinic.

5. Access to the living systems of the community for reintegra-
tion of discharged mental patients into naturally occurring
support systems of the community.

All but 15 *espiritistas* and *santero(a)s* interviewed by the ICSS project
in Newark welcome such cooperative efforts. This strategy of reciprocal consultation and referral within already existing linkages would not
co-opt or subordinate the folk healer to the orthodox system and it
would permit the orthodox practitioner the degree of supervision and
control over the services provided his/her own patients to satisfy ethical
considerations.

But, what is possible and appropriate in the Puerto Rican community cannot be generalized to other communities and other "spiritual" beliefs and practitioners. The *espiritistas'* practices are the pro-
totype of what I have called elsewhere (Garrison, 1978) "natural network therapy," recommending this as the modality of care delivery
which fits naturally and congenially into the habitual patterns of help-
seeking, help-giving, and help-receiving in the Puerto Rican community. These patterns include neighborhood-based walk-in services, a
flexible combination of individual, group, family and network therapies, with open groups and attendance on the basis of felt need,
emphasis on role playing and psychodramatic techniques, with clinicians participating in the informal social organization and communication networks of the community.[17] The Puerto Rican folk practices are
distinctive in this style of delivery. The related belief systems in general
American white culture (spiritualism) and in black American culture
("spiritual" or "spiritualist" counselors and churches) have evolved
with very different styles of help-seeking, help-giving, help-receiving,
and relationships to orthodox health care. The modalities, the techniques, the rules of confidentiality, and the attitudes toward professional care are different, despite similar beliefs in "spiritual" forces.
This point will be elaborated in future publications, but, for example:
Black

and white American spiritual counselors do not draw their clientele primarily from the immediate neighborhood, services are provided by appointment, and the "spiritual working" of deeply personal matters within an open group, as in *Espiritismo*, is not done. The black American spiritual practices tend to be strictly one-to-one and "secret," and clients prefer to go outside of their local neighborhoods for greater anonymity and confidentiality. The mainstream American practices of "spiritualism" are a counterculture phenomenon with the same basic culture patterns as those of the professional care system but with an oppositional philosophy. The three layers of communication of mediums, as self, as good spirit, and as bad spirit, and the "mirroring" techniques in which the spirit speaks *for* rather than *to* the client, appear unique to the Hispanic practices among those studied. These differences in healing practices based on similar beliefs between different groups reflect variations in the subcultures which are repeated throughout many spheres of life, including but not limited to the folk-healing beliefs and practices themselves.

The greatest potential benefit to the orthodox mental health care system from linkage with these folk practitioners is the identification of these naturally occurring support system patterns within subculturally distinct communities, thus permitting the better adaptation of the mental health care delivery system to the life of the community and the adoption of those professional techniques and modalities of patient care that are most congenial, acceptable and, therefore, probably effective, in that culture.

FOOTNOTES

1. This project is supported by U.S. Public Health Service Grant No. 1R01 MH28467, to the College of Medicine and Dentistry of New Jersey, New Jersey Medical School, Newark, N.J., Vivian Garrison, Ph.D., Principal Investigator (September 1, 1976–August 31, 1981).
2. U.S. Public Health Service Grant No. 1 R01 MH22563, "Folk Healers and Community Mental Health Programming," to Columbia University, Department of Anthropology, New York, N.Y., Vivian Garrison, Ph.D. and Alexander Alland, Ph.D., Co-Principal Investigators (October 1, 1972–December 31, 1976). That research and demonstration project was located by collaborative arrangement in the Tremont Crisis Center of Bronx State Hospital and Albert Einstein College of Medicine under Drs. Israel Zwerling and Edward T. Hornich.

3. I was myself living in the community at the time and participated in these events as well as documenting them through
   observations and formal and informal interviews. All group
   sessions in the *centro* and many private consultations were
   also tape recorded. The principal parties in this episode were
   also interviewed using the Current and Past Psychiatric Status Schedule (CAPPS) (Endicott and Spitzer, 1972) and
   psychiatric opinions of each, together with projected professional treatment plans, were provided by Dr. Gladys Egri,
   Clinical Associate Professor of Psychiatry, Columbia University, College of Physicians and Surgeons. For reasons of
   confidentiality and anonymity these opinions are not reported explicitly here, but I have drawn upon them heavily
   in my description of the case histories. My thanks to Dr. Egri
   and also to Margaret Beels, M.S.W., who read and commented upon an earlier version of this manuscript. My most
   heartfelt thanks also to Loreta Colon, *Espiritista* and *Iyalocha,*
   who has been my "teacher" *(maestra)* in *Espiritismo* and godmother *(madrina)* in *Santería* since I began these studies in
   1965. For more detailed discussion of the methods, and the
   quantitative results of this study see Garrison, 1977b.
4. All names are pseudonyms and identifying features have
   been altered to obscure identities from third parties without
   distorting the facts of the case. Fully informed consent has
   been obtained from all parties for the publication of their
   case histories, anonymously. My utmost thanks to all of
   them, although they must remain anonymous.
5. It is not clear whether these seizures are organically based or
   are the more common *"ataque de nervios"* (nervous attack),
   usually an hysterical mechanism.
6. *"Causa"* in *Espiritismo* means "cause" literally, or the etiology
   of the problem. *"Causas,"* are of two kinds: "material," or
   natural, and "spiritual," or immaterial. In the spiritual sense,
   "causa" also refers specifically to the molesting spirit that is
   the cause of the problem. Terms like this from *Espiritismo*
   that are not adequately rendered in English translation will
   be left in Spanish in the text.
7. These spirits are "with" the person and specific to that one
   person. They may be inside or outside, close or far away, at
   different times, but the issue of whether the impulses,
   thoughts, feelings and behavior that they represent be located *inside* the individual *or outside* is a major concern in
   American psychologies and psychotherapies which is
   irrelevant in *Espiritismo.*

8. *"Fluidos"* is literally translatable as "fluids," but in *Espiritismo* it means both the "ectoplasm" of the spirit and the sensations one feels from the presence of a spirit. In this particular context, it means the sensations of Consuelo's own spirit and might best be translated by the vernacular "vibes."

9. *Evidencias,* or evidences, refer generally to all spiritual evidence for the existence of spirits or spiritual causation, and also specifically to the visualizations of the spiritual conditions that mediums "see."

10. The implication in *Espiritismo* is that these spirits want Dolores to be like them or that they give her the symptoms and characteristics they had before their deaths. They have to be "educated" that they are "dead" and can no longer experience these pains.

11. All adolescents and nearly half of all diagnosed spiritually in this centro over a six-month period were said to be "in development."

12. As president of the *centro* Rosa is also the director of the psychodramatic enactments that take place there, and there is ample evidence in the many case histories collected from her practice that she clearly postpones the "working of the spirits" until such time as the person is readied to receive the "communications" of the "spirits."

13. An orthodox psychotherapist might consider this establishment of a fictitious mother–daughter relationship between the healer and the client as an institutionalization of the transference and a reinforcement of dependency and, therefore, contraindicated. But, it is very interesting to note that the *espiritistas* can and do offer themselves as continuously available upon demand to all clients and they, nonetheless, do not have caseloads that grow beyond bounds. In Rosa's *centro* no one is permitted to stay around the *centro* exclusively in the sick role. Once Rosa has "cured" them of whatever it was they come complaining about, they are expected to either consider themselves "cured" and not in need of spiritual help until the next crisis, or, if they continue to come to the *centro*, they are expected to "develop faculties," and assist in the "working" of others with "whatever they have to give."

14. There are many Hispanic paraprofessionals, and some professionals as well, who have such unofficial collaborative and reciprocal referral relationships with folk practitioners. Such relationships have been formalized and institutionalized in the Lincoln Community Mental Health Center pro-

gram (Ruiz, 1976) where Puerto Rican community mental health workers who were also spiritist believers, were officially assigned to act in this liaison role as part of their agency duties.

15. Gerald Caplan defined "support systems" as "continuing social aggregates (namely, continuing interactions with another individual, a network, a group, or an organization) that provide individuals with opportunities for feedback about themselves and for validation of their expectations about others, which may offset deficiencies in those communications within the larger community context." (Caplan, 1974, 1976, p. 19) "Such support," he continued, "may be of a continuing nature or intermittent and short-term and may be utilized from time to time by the individual in the event of an acute need or crisis. Both enduring and short-term supports are likely to consist of three elements: (a) the significant others help the individual mobilize his psychological resources and master his emotional burdens; (b) they share his tasks; and (c) they provide him with extra supplies of money, materials, tools, skills, and cognitive guidance to improve his handling of his situation." (Caplan, 1974, pp. 5–6; 1976, p. 20) In his usage "a family," "a church," "a network" or "a folk healing group" is "a support system." In my usage here and elsewhere (Garrison, 1978, p. 562), the "support system" is defined differently. Social structure, with any elements, and the functions of "support" are conceived separately and there is no assumption that "support" is necessarily clinically positive as for example, with the family system of a schizophrenic, the rescuers and drinking buddies of an alcoholic, or the "madam," "pimp" and "johns" in the social network of a prostitute, all of whom may provide support to an individual to reinforce and maintain a psychopathological life style.

The "social network" is a structural concept defined, following Kapferer (1969, p. 182) as " . . . the direct links radiating from a particular Ego to other individuals, and the links which connect those individuals who are directly tied to Ego, to one another." In this network, the elements are individuals who may be family members, neighbors, friends, voluntary association members, agency representatives, psychotherapists, or any other individual with whom Ego has contacts, and the linkages or functions are interactions, which may or may not be "supportive." "Support" for the individual Ego within this network is conceived as any interaction conforming to those three "support" categories delineated by Caplan, and is operationally defined as: those relationships in which ego reports *(1)* that he or she can count on the person (or institution or agency) for financial help, help with household tasks, child care, or help when ill (instrumental support); *(2)* that he or she discusses problems with or confides in that person (cognitive guidance and affective support); or *(3)* that he or she seeks that person's help in times of distress (crisis support).

16.   Pedro Rodriguez, M.D. was the psychiatrist who did these assessments in the Hispanic communities. Eugenia Curet, M.S.W., Ana Hernandez, B.A., Judith Podell, B.A., and I were the ethnographic field workers and "culture specialists" in the Hispanic communities and clinic.

17.   This style of service delivery was developed as the most amenable and appropriate, independent of the folk healer example, for the low-income black and Puerto Rican community of the South Bronx in the early 1960s by the Lincoln Hospital Mental Health Services (Peck et al., 1966), later replaced by a community mental health center program which appears to me less well adapted to the community.

REFERENCES

Abad, V. and Boyce, E. Issues in psychiatric evaluations of Puerto Ricans: A socio-cultural perspective. *Journal of Operational Psychiatry*, 1979, *10* (1), 28–39.

Abad, V., Ramos, J., and Boyce, E. A model for the delivery of mental health services to Spanish-speaking minorities. *American Journal of Orthopsychiatry*, 1974, *44* (4), 584–595.

Baer, H. A. Black spiritual churches: The role of a neglected religious movement. Paper delivered at the American Anthropological Association Annual Meeting, November 27–December 1, 1979, Cincinnati, Ohio.

Baer, H. A. Black spiritual churches: A neglected socio-religious category. *Phylon: Atlantic University Journal of Race and Culture* (forthcoming).

Bannerman, R. H. WHO's programme. World health, November 16–17. Reprinted in WHO's programme in traditional medicine, *WHO Chronicle*, 1977, *31* (11), 427–428.

Bellak, L., Hurvich, M., and Godiman, H. K. *Ego functions in schizophrenics, neurotics, and normals.* New York: John Wiley & Sons, 1973.

Bergman, R. L. A school for medicine men. *American Journal of Psychiatry*, 1973, *130* (6), 663–666.

Bibeau, G. The world health organization in encounter with African traditional medicine: Theoretical conceptions and practical strategies, in Ademu-wagen, Z. A., Ayoade, J. A. A., Harrison, I. E., and Warren, D. M., eds. *African therapeutic systems.* Waltham, Mass.: African Studies Association, Crossroads Press, 1979, 182–186.

Caplan, G. *Support systems and community mental health: Lectures on concept development.* New York: Behavioral Publications, 1974.

Caplan, G. Introduction and overview, in Caplan, G. and Killilea, M., eds. *Support systems and mutual help: Multidisciplinary explorations.* New York: Grune and Stratton, 1976.

Endicott, J. and Spitzer, R. L. Current and past psychopathology scales (CAPPS): Rationale, reliability and validity. *Archives of General Psychiatry,* 1972, *27,* 678–687.

Fields, S. Folk healing for the wounded spirit and psychiatry and the melting pot myth. *Innovations,* 1976, *3* (1), 2–24.

Garrison, V. The "Puerto Rican syndrome" in Psychiatry and *Espiritismo,* in Crapanzano, V. and Garrison, V., eds. *Case studies in spirit possession.* New York: John Wiley, 1977a, pp. 383–449.

Garrison, V. Doctor, *espiritista* or psychiatrist? Health-seeking behavior in a Puerto Rican neighborhood of New York City. *Medical Anthropology,* 1977b, *1* (2), 65–191.

Garrison, V. Support systems of schizophrenic and nonschizophrenic Puerto Rican migrant women in New York City. *Schizophrenia Bulletin,* 1978, *4* (4), 561–596.

Garrison, V. and Podell. J. A practicable "community support systems assessment" for inclusion in standard clinical interviews. Paper prepared for Conference on Stress, Social Support, and Schizophrenia, National Institute of Mental Health, Burlington, Vt., September 24–25, 1979. (ICSS Working Paper #12).

Hall, A. L. and Bourne, P. G. Indigenous therapists in a southern black urban community. *Archives of General Psychiatry,* 1973, *28,* 137–142.

Harwood, A. *Rx: Spiritist as needed.* New York: Wiley, 1977.

Jilek, W. G. From crazy witch doctor to auxiliary psychotherapist—the changing image of the medicine man. *Psychiatria Clinica,* 1971, *4,* 200–220.

Jordan, W. C. Voodoo medicine, in Williams, R. A., ed. *Textbook of black-related diseases.* New York: McGraw-Hill, Blackston Publication, 1975, pp. 715–738.

Kapferer, B. Norms and the manipulation of relations in work situations, in Mitchell, J. C., ed. *Social networks in urban situations.* Manchester: Manchester University Press, 1969, pp. 181–244.

Kleinman, A. M. Concepts and a model for the comparison of medical systems as cultural systems. *Culture, Medicine and Psychiatry,* 1978, *2* (3), 85–93.

Koss, J. Therapeutic aspects of Puerto Rican cult practices. *Psychiatry,* 1975, *38,* 160–171.

Koss, J. Therapist-spiritist training project in Puerto Rico. U.S. Public Health

Service Grant No. MH 14310–02 (July 1, 1977–June 30, 1980), J. Koss, Ph.D., Principal Investigator.

Koss, J. Social process, healing, and self-defeat among Puerto Rican spiritists. *American Ethnologist*, 1977, *4* (3), 453–469.

Leslie, C. M., ed. *Asian medical systems*. Berkeley: University of California Press, 1976.

Lubchansky, I., Egri, G., and Stokes, J. Puerto Rican spiritualists view mental illness: The faith healer as a paraprofessional. *American Journal of Psychiatry*, 1970, *127* (3), 312–321.

Mayer, A. C. The significance of quasi-groups in the study of complex societies, in Banton, M., ed. *The social anthropology of complex societies*. London: Tavistock, 1966, pp. 87–122.

McGuire, M. *Baltimore Catechism No. 2 with special prayer, mass and confirmation sections*. New York: Benziger Brothers, 1962.

Osborne, O. H. The Yoruba village as a therapeutic community. *Journal of Health and Social Behavior*, 1969, *10* (3), 187–200.

Peck, H. B., Kaplan, S. R., and Roman, M. Prevention, treatment and social action: A strategy of intervention in a disadvantaged urban area. *American Journal of Orthopsychiatry*, 1966, *36* (1), 57–59.

President's Commission on Mental Health. Task panel report vol. II, Community support systems. Washington, D.C.: Superintendent of Documents, Government Printing Office, 1978, pp. 168–179.

Press, I. Problems in the definition and classification of medical systems. *Social Science and Medicine*, 1980, *14B* (1).

Prince, R. Variations in psychotherapeutic procedures, in Triandis, H. C. and Draguns, J. G., eds. *Handbook of cross-cultural psychology*. Boston: Alleyn and Bacon, 1980, Vol. VI.

Rogler, L. and Hollingshead, A. B. The Puerto Rican spiritualist as psychiatrist. *American Journal of Sociology*, 1961, *67*, 17–21.

Rogler, L. and Hollingshead, A. B. *Trapped: Families and schizophrenia*. New York: John Wiley, 1965, pp. 243–260.

Ruiz, P. Folk healers as associate therapist, in Masserman, J. H., ed. *Current Psychiatric Therapies*, Vol. 16. New York: Grune and Stratton, 1976.

Sandoval, M. *Santería* as a mental health care system: A historical overview. *Social Science and Medicine*, 1979, *13* (2), 137–152.

Scott, C. S. Health and healing practices among five ethnic groups in Miami, Florida, in Bauwens, E. E., ed. *The anthropology of health*. St. Louis, Mo.: C. V. Mosby, 1974, pp. 61–70.

Singer, P., ed. Introduction: From anthropology and medicine to "therapy" and neo-colonialism. Special issue: Traditional healing: New science or new colonialism? *The Conch*, 1976, pp. 1–25.

Snow, L. F. Sorcerers, saints and charlatans: Black folk healers in urban America. *Culture Medicine and Psychiatry*, 1979, pp. 69–106.

Thomas, C. S. and Garrison, V. A general systems view of community mental health, in Bellak, L. and Barten, H., eds. *Progress in community mental health.* New York: Brunner/Mazel, 1975, pp. 265–332.

Torrey, E. F. *The mind game: Witchdoctors and psychiatrists.* New York: Emerson-Hall, 1972.

Weidman, H. H. *Miami health ecology project report,* Vol. I. A statement of ethnicity and health. Miami: University of Miami (Xerox, 1978).

Weidman, H. H. The transcultural view: Prerequisites to interethnic (intercultural) communication in medicine. *Social Science and Medicine,* 1979, *13* (2), 85–87.

Chapter 4

COMMUNITY SUPPORT SYSTEMS

An Alternative Approach to Mental Health Service Delivery

Arthur J. Naparstek, Ph.D.
David E. Biegel, L.C.S.W.

Naparstek and Biegel have studied a selected sample of ethnic neighborhoods and emphasize the importance of these neighborhoods as a source of support for its residents. The authors provide evidence that social class and cultural aspects do affect the mental health status and the use of services in the community. The authors effectively argue for the creation of community support systems developed through a partnership between lay and professional people.

Through the use of vignettes, Naparstek and Biegel focus on the importance, the uniqueness, and the strength of a community-based support system in operation. They outline an innovative capacity-building model which integrates lay and professional services within a community for effective delivery.

COMMUNITY SUPPORT SYSTEMS—ROLE AND EFFECTIVENESS

It has finally dawned upon America, the land of good and plenty, that its resources—physical and human—might not be endless. As budgets are tightening, demands are increasing for cost-effective initiatives to meet society's needs. The energy crisis has stimulated new standards for fuel-efficient automobiles and carpools, and turned down (or up) thermostats. In the fields of mental health and human service, the pioneer spirit of neighbor helping neighbor has been discovered—again. Self-help is in vogue.

Americans have been involved in mutual-aid programs since the first urban communities were founded here, but the government has only recently "rediscovered" the self-help approach. Reports of the President's Commission on Mental Health and the National Commissions on Neighborhoods, and the President's Urban Policy Message, paid tribute to the potential of the self-help impulse in addressing human and community problems in American cities. This recognition is generally welcomed, but the prospect of the government embracing and involving itself wholesale in informal, nonprofessional urban community support systems ought to be regarded with caution.

If the government studies self-help programs and organizations with an eye to learning how they operate and why they are effective— then uses these data to develop policy initiatives that will enhance community support systems and link them productively with public and private programs—all well and good. If, however, self-help programs and groups are viewed as vehicles for replacing public monies sliced from tight budgets, then we will find that the self-help movement is moving backward, not progressing.

Community support systems are, in many ways, fragile entities. Government intervention in their operations—even if well-intentioned—might seriously undermine the basic conditions and premises that make them work so well. A thoughtful approach to the potential role of community support systems in the delivery of mental health and human services[1] should involve:

1. comprehension of the nature of community support systems and their operations;
2. evaluation of the critical issues in the delivery of mental health services today;
3. exploration of the kinds of linkages which might mutually benefit community support systems, on the one hand, and professional mental health delivery systems, on the other; and
4. the framing of public policy initiatives which would strengthen community support systems and promote appropriate linkages between them and professional delivery systems.

NATURE AND OPERATION OF COMMUNITY SUPPORT SYSTEMS

The functioning parts of a community support system might include:

the retired schoolteacher to whom elderly neighbors turn for
help and advice when their social security checks are late,

the ethnic organization that helps a middle-aged couple cope
with strains caused by value conflicts with their teenaged children,

the community association that sets up a telephone crisis hotline
for its neighborhood,

the luncheonette waitress whom customers talk to about their
marital problems,

the older lady who took in a 14-year-old girl after she had been
thrown out by her family,

the clergyman parishioners go to with their family problems, and

the retired practical nurse who helps a neighbor care for an aged
parent

In a pluralistic society, people seek help, solve problems and meet
their needs in varying ways. Family, friends, neighbors, co-workers,
clergy, neighborhood organizations, and mutual-aid groups can provide meaningful assistance in times of need. All of these helping
entities are encompassed by the term "Community Support System."

Community support systems serve a preventive function by contributing to an individual's sense of well-being and competent functioning. They can assist in reducing the negative consequences of
stressful life events. Community support systems can be especially
important for the chronically mentally ill, who need assistance in
recovering from the isolation of institutional life.

Community support systems include both person-to-person and
organizational support. Person-to-person caregiving efforts have
usually developed without professional support or assistance. Most
organizational forms of community support systems, such as mutual
aid groups and neighborhood organizations, have similarly developed
without professional intervention. Support systems are also natural in
the sense that they are ongoing and not formally organized. Some
forms of support systems develop in response to a specific societal
problem or in response to the lack of professional services to address a
particular problem. The problem of divorce, for example, has led to
support groups for the divorced.

Community support systems serve all of us to some degree, and in
different ways. More specifically, they serve many population groups
which are unable or unwilling to seek professional help, or for whom
professional services are currently lacking. These include ethnic and
racial minorities, women, and the aged. Community support systems
offer help in a culturally acceptable manner without attendant stigma
or loss of pride. The individuals seeking help need not identify them-

selves as having a problem, being weak, or sick or being a client or patient, as would be necessary when seeking professional help.

Much research testifies to the importance of these support systems (Litwak, 1961; Breton, 1964; Slater, 1970; Glazer, 1971; Warren, 1977; Caplan, 1974; and Collins and Pancoast, 1976). Donald Warren (1977) states that strengthening these support systems can help an individual (1) gain a sense of control over one's life, (2) reduce alienation from society, (3) gain a capacity to solve new problems, and (4) maintain the motivation to overcome the handicaps and frustrations of modern society.

There is strong evidence that the availability of social supports in a community acts as a buffer in times of crisis, enabling people to cope and adapt to change (Warren, 1977; Caplan and Killilea, 1976). Even superficial links with neighbors can add up to a significant support system directly affecting treatment outcomes for people in crisis.

Collins and Pancoast (1976) review numerous studies of informal caregivers and indicate their tremendous potential in mental health and human services as a vital bridge between the individual, the environment and the service professional. These informal counterparts to organized social services carry the largest part of the service load in many service areas. Too often, they observe, service professionals are trained to focus exclusively on problems that require professional help, ignoring the informal supportive network. Lee (1969) reported on the importance of informal social networks in finding and selecting an abortionist. Caplan and Killilea (1976) discussed the work of Traunstein and Killilea, who found that many people in an upper New York State community received service from their peers which paralleled, complemented, and, in many instances, competed with the professional service network. Snyder (1971) reported his findings of the importance of community gatekeepers to crisis management. Naparstek et al. (1977) documented the important helping services being provided in urban ethnic communities by clergy, neighborhood leaders and natural helpers. Sarason et al. (1977) discussed the importance of kin family networks in the lives of the increasing numbers of single, widowed and divorced individuals in society. Barbarin, Mitchell, and Hurley (unpublished paper) found that active citizens maintained linkages to a variety of both formal and informal resource networks and were able to respond competently to problem situations with an impressive number and variety of solutions utilizing both systems.

Other studies have focused on neighborhoods as an important context for the operation of support systems. Berger and Neuhaus (1977) discussed the importance of "mediating structures," such as the neighborhood, church and family, which operate between individuals in their private lives and the large institutions of public life. They stated that the neighborhood should be seen as a key structure and argued that service programs ought to be developed through these relevant mediating institutions. People, working in small groups around concerns of the neighborhood, strengthen both their own internal networks and the mediating institutions, making it possible to link themselves to other systems for solving mutual problems (Naparstek, 1976; Doughton, 1976; Berger and Neuhaus, 1977).

Community support systems comprise an important component of the strength and resources often found in neighborhoods. Our own research, the Neighborhood and Family Services Project, with data from two urban ethnic communities, show that there are impressive numbers of professional and lay (family, friends, neighbors, etc.) community helpers.[2] Many of these helpers live in the neighborhoods they serve and have done so for years. They express generally positive feelings about these neighborhoods, despite the existence of many community issues and problems. Our data also show that lay helpers express a strong sense of community pride and, in turn, are highly regarded and trusted by community residents. Residents, we have learned, prefer to take care of their own problems if they can, without seeking professional assistance. They accept the assistance and support of trusted lay helpers. Lay helpers, on the other hand, recognize the limits of their areas of expertise and indicated that outside their own areas of competence, they value the resources of mental health professionals. The positive involvement of the lay helpers in the neighborhoods, the inclination of the community residents toward self-help, the large number and availability of lay helpers, the trust afforded to these informal caregivers and the preference for the services of lay help, emphasize the importance of these support systems. But none of this is meant to suggest that professional services are not important, or that community support systems can meet all needs. Quite the opposite is true. Both systems are important. To be fully effective, they should be linked to each other.

The effectivenes of community support systems can be gauged by the critical role they play in addressing the mental health and human services problems of fragmentation, lack of accessibility, and lack of accountability. Vignettes from the author's Neighborhood and Family Services Project explain their operation.

A Community Support Systems Approach Can Reach Populations in Need of Assistance Unwilling or Unable to Seek Professional Help.

Through a community-sponsored research process, we became aware that large numbers of ethnic working-class women on the south side of Milwaukee were living alone. Many of these women were divorced or widowed, and considered at high risk for developing mental health problems. Ethnic working-class women do not traditionally seek help from mental health centers. Neither do they tend to participate in organized self-help groups. This is a population that the mental health community does not know how to reach. As a result, these women are largely underserved, except in psychiatric emergencies.

When our project began, there were no support groups for the divorced or widowed on the south side. The local mental health center could not be approached for assistance for fear a support group started in conjunction with a mental health center would be seen as stigmatizing the population. Instead, our local community organization approached a local clergyman and secured the names of a dozen widowed members of his parish. The widows were approached by a community organizer as to their needs and interest for a support group. The widows expressed reluctance. When they found out, however, that their pastor was supporting the program, they changed their minds and came to a meeting. Separate community-wide support groups for widows with children, widows without children, and the divorced involving well over 100 persons have since sprung from this first organizational meeting of four widows.

By working through community networks of clergy and neighborhood organizations, ethnic working-class women became involved in self-help efforts sponsored under the aegis of the community. The groups are organized around their needs and interests. Once the groups felt confident enough, they approached professionals for assistance. Professionals became advisors to a community-directed process, a reversal of the normal professional role. To be effective, the initial organizing effort had to come from the community, not the professional sector.

In Baltimore, a 72-year-old feebleminded man was evicted from his apartment shortly before Thanksgiving Day for owing $200 in rent. Neighbors called the Neighborhood Hotline for help. A number of agencies were contacted, but immediate help was not forthcoming. There was no single agency which was willing or able to handle the man's problem. A lay helper swung into action. She called the landlord and told him forcefully that he had been wrong to evict the tenant; she pointed out a number of agencies that could have been called for assistance. She complained of the victim's possessions having been put out on the street. The landlord replied that she should not worry since the tenant had a few possessions anyway, and what he did have was not worth much. The community helper became incensed, informing the landlord that what the tenant did have meant a great deal to him because he treasured his possessions. The landlord took the tenant back in, and undoubtedly suffered from pangs of conscience on Thanksgiving Day. The community helper, in turn, agreed to help the landlord obtain professional help for his tenant.

A Community Support Systems Approach Is Built Upon the Strengths, Not Weaknesses of the Community.

On the south side of Milwaukee, Wisconsin, a federally funded community mental health center had for several years been aware of problems of family communication in the neighborhood. The center had tried unsuccessfully to organize family communication seminars as a means of addressing this issue, lacking community access and support. The tightly knit proud community on the south side of Milwaukee was unwilling to let a professional agency define their problems. Through the Neighborhood and Family Services Project, community residents collected and analyzed for themselves relevant data on community strength and needs. They themselves identified family communications as a problem. They decided to build a program based on community strength and utilizing existing neighborhood helpers. Professionals were brought in as advisors to the community-directed planning process. As a result, a series of very successful, well-attended, family communication workshops were held in the community.

A Community Support Systems Approach Builds Upon the Unique Ability of Community Residents to Know What Will "Work" in Their Community.

In Baltimore, a Community Health Education Network was formed to promote mental and physical health. The mental health committee of the network decided that a four-part workshop series on "stress" would be desirable. They contacted the director of a local community psychiatry program about staffing the workshops. The director, a psychiatrist, agreed to work with the community group. He had definite ideas about how the workshop should be run, and wanted the focus narrowed to one particular kind of stress, such as occupational or marital. He wanted the entire four-part workshop preplanned. Community members disagreed; they felt that more flexibility was needed. After some discussion, the psychiatrist decided to "wing it." He agreed to a planning meeting before each workshop session to review the last session and plan the next. He also agreed that the workshop would indeed focus on all aspects of stress.

Community members distributed flyers for the workhop, illustrated with little bugs, which read, "What's bugging you? Come to the Stress Workshop!" A potluck dinner preceded each session. Up to 70 individuals attended individual sessions. Results of a written evaluation form after the last session were extremely positive.

The principal point here is that the psychiatrist's main concern was with the format of the workshop for greatest effectiveness, viewed from professional standards. The community's principal concern was getting people to attend, feel relaxed, and talk about their problems. The workshop surpassed the community's wildest hopes. Residents who attended have subsequently told planning committee members that they now feel it is "safe" to talk about stress and problems. They have commented that "the shrink was okay" and "psychiatrists aren't bad." The psychiatrist, however, while pleased, still isn't sure how to evaluate the workshop. His idea of an effective workshop would not have worked in southeast Baltimore at the present time. It would have been regarded as too formal and too professional by the residents of this working class community, who would simply not have attended.

A Community Support Systems Approach Can Enhance Accountabilty, Sometimes in Interesting Ways.

In Baltimore, a dozen elderly residents frantically came to the front door of a lay helper well known for her advocacy skills. Their social security checks had not arrived that morning. Since the social security check was their only income, they did not know what to do and were very frightened. They pleaded with the neighborhood helper to "call somebody up and do something." This woman, 65 years old herself and dependent on her social security check, was also nervous, but she hid her anxiety from the group. She called the local post office to complain. She was told that the mailman had left early in the morning with the social security checks. Since it was already 2:00 P.M. when she called, she pressed the post office to track down the lost mailman. Then she explained the situation to her elderly neighbors and urged them to go back to their houses and wait. They refused and stayed at her doorstep. A short while later, the mailman arrived, having been roused from a local drinking establishment. He found an angry group of social security recipients, shouting out their names and demanding their checks. Doubtlessly it was an accountability experience he will never forget.

Creating Linkages Between Community Support Systems and Mental Health and Human Service Programs Can Reduce Fragmentation of Services and Provide Help in a More Effective Way.

In Baltimore, a telephone crisis hotline, run by neighborhood residents, was established to help institutionalize the natural work of neighborhood helpers. Because the hotline is staffed by neighborhood helpers and not professionals, it reaches some individuals who would not seek professional help.

One day a former mental patient called the hotline and threatened to kill himself. The hotline volunteer did everything she could to keep him talking. After a few minutes, she asked him if he were dressed. When he said he was not, she told him to get dressed right away and promised to call him back in five minutes. In those five minutes, she made calls to the crisis clinic at a local hospital and arranged for a trained professional to go to the man's house and take him to a local psychiatric clinic for immediate help. The hotline volunteer was quick, perceptive, competent, and effective because she knew all the various resources in the community, and she personally knew professinals at the crisis clinic and could call them directly—not an easy feat when dealing with a large hospital bureaucracy. This process works when lay helpers and mental health professionals work in tandem to assist people in times of crisis. The expertise of the lay helper, coupled with the resources and accessibility of the community hotline, was responsible for preventing a suicide.

Also in Baltimore, an elderly gentleman in poor health, on crutches, was caring for his invalid wife at home. He could not bear to see her sent to a nursing home, so he began selling their household belongings in order to pay for nursing care for his wife in his home. (It is ironical that medical insurance would cover the cost of "institutional" care in a nursing home, but not home care.) After his wife died, government authorities wanted the man removed to a nursing home since he required too much assistance to live at home. At this point, the neighborhood helping network sprang into action. Through the Neighborhood and Family Services Project Hotline, a community helper learned of the issue. She contacted neighbors of the man and mobilized a coordinated, accountable, unfragmented helping system of community helpers to aid him. As a result, he is still living in his home, with reliable neighbors doing the necessary grocery shopping, cooking, cleaning, and house maintenance to enable him to stay in the community.

Professional services now serve as an important backup to the efforts of these community helpers. Only through the efforts of both the community support system in the neighborhood and professional services was the man able to remain in his community.

Creating Linkages Between Community Support Systems and Mental Health and Human Service Professionals Can Help Reinforce the Work of Lay Helpers and Demystify the Role of Professionals.

In Baltimore, a clergy/agency/community seminar attracted over 80 persons. Part of the seminar involved small mixed groups of clergy, agency, and community helpers meeting to explore the strengths and resources of each helping group. At a debriefing meeting of the organizing committee after the seminar, a clergyman remarked that the community helpers learned for the first time that professionals did not have all the answers either.. As a result, they felt encouraged and better able to go out and help people. In all previous dealings with professionals, these community helpers had felt "one down." At the seminar, however, they had equal status with the professionals, and this enabled them to see through the mirage of professional omnipotence!

These examples graphically demonstrate the importance of community support systems in situations where professionals alone could not hope to be successful. The data from our Neighborhood and Family Services Project shows that professionals are often unaware of the degree and scope of the lay helping systems described above and do not recognize or interact significantly with lay helpers. Furthermore, lay helpers are often unaware of other lay helpers and the contributions that the lay helping network as a whole makes to mental health service delivery. They are also not fully aware of professional resources. While lay helpers are more aware of problems in the community than professionals, they do indicate a lack of knowledge about the problems of some specific population groups. At the same time, our research findings show low resident utilization of professional services and high indications that people do not know where to turn for help, either within the lay or the professional helping systems.

It is clear that for the support systems to be most effective, they need to be linked with professionals. In fact, such linkages are already partly operational in many communities although there are often significant obstacles that make it difficult for professional and community helpers to work together.

Promoting Partnerships Between Mental Health Services and Community Support Systems

Incipient networks, both lay and professional, are in place in many urban communities. Experiences of the University of Southern California's Neighborhood and Family Services Project, as well as other studies, demonstrate potential for the development of an integrated lay and professonal service delivery system. Our data reveal that our pilot neighborhoods in Baltimore and Milwaukee are very stable. Residents express strong positive neighborhood attachment and wholehearted approval of self-help values. An established community support system in either community would not collapse easily. Network-building efforts in such communities tend to be self-reinforcing and self-generating. Since lay helpers have recognized the importance of professional services, there is strong potential for productive linkages with the professional network.

Professionals working in these communities express generally positive attitudes toward the neighborhoods they serve. This suggests that they, too, regard the neighborhood as a positive environment for social interaction, and that they are optimistic about future potential. Professionals who harbored doubts about neighborhood possibilities would not be likely to wish to cooperate with community efforts to create an integrated helping network. In fact, professionals in the two pilot communities have begun to participate in activities of the local community organizations. They evince sympathy with the need to provide more convenient services, and they express identical views with residents on the identification of critical community problems. All this suggests strong potential for development of successful partnerships between professional and lay helpers.

The ongoing dialogue which would undoubtedly ensue from such linkages would enable members of each network to identify service gaps, duplications, and opportunities for more coordination. In the communities we studied, there seemed to be at least one helping network, lay or professional, which had knowledge of each problem or each at-risk population group, and resources for appropriate intervention. Development of an integrated, coordinated network system would mean that knowledgeable groups could influence and educate groups which were less aware. A self-correction mechanism would come into operation, so that lay and professional helpers could come to understand how each defined problems and how each chose appropriate resources.

Situations arise in which professionals, lay helpers, and community residents evaluate some mental health problems differently (see Barbarin, Mitchell, and Hurley, unpublished paper). When lay helpers assessed situations as nonpsychiatric, they preferred to rely on family, clergy, or other community helping resources. Professionals tended to refer clients to psychiatrists in instances which the residents regarded as nonpsychiatric (Naparstek, Biegel, et al., 1979). The clients were then unlikely to follow through on recommended treatment. If the professionals had access to supportive lay helping networks which could complement or endorse their recommendations, the follow-through would be more likely to occur. The partnership approach has an additional dividend: intervention through a lay network can reduce and frequently eliminate, the stigma attached to seeking and receiving mental health service and treatment in urban, ethnic neighborhoods. When school-behavior problems arise in a community, for instance, teens and their parents who need help are not likely to feel stigmatized if they begin with a family life education workshop held at the local school and sponsored by a community association.

Strong potential for productive lay and professional partnerships exists, but so do serious obstacles arising from biases and from attitudinal and value differences. Both professionals and community helpers, because they tend to focus on specific population groups and services, may have a restricted view of community needs. Mental health and human service professionals may think that they have "all the answers," all the expertise, and all the skill necessary to help people in need. They may underestimate the assistance that untrained community residents can provide. By these observations, we do not mean to denigrate professionals: they have valuable skills and assets. Unfortunately, the professionals, by themselves, may not be able to reach many people who would never, for reasons of pride or privacy, go to a professional for help. In addition, professionals are not likely to be fully aware of community values, resources and networks that are already providing support to persons in need in their own way. It takes little imagination to recognize that the mental health and human service needs of any urban community are so tremendous that if lay community workers stopped helping people, professional systems would soon become overloaded.

Professionals and lay helpers have serious problems communicating with one another. Professionals tend to aggregate needs of individuals and to speak about "at risk population groups" and "underserved areas." They utilize statistics, surveys, needs assessments, etc. Community helpers speak about individuals: John Brown, the retired man down the block who needs help taking care of his wife; Ann Black, the woman with three children, who cannot seem to cope. Community helpers cannot understand why a client is not "eligible" for services— he has problems, does he not? Professionals, with their caseloads, waiting lists, rules, and regulations, may have less flexibility than community workers. They may not be able to give the kind of help they would like to give. The lay helpers, on the other hand, sometimes think that they are the *only* ones who really care about people, the *only* ones who really want to help. They are skeptical about professionals' motives. Professionals just work from 9–5 P.M., they say, while they are on call all the time.

Differences in education, training, and class and ethnic background further complicate lay–professional relationships. Indeed, the two groups seem to speak to each other in different languages. The lay workers discuss needs on an intuitive or "gut" level, in colloquial terms. The professionals, who are most comfortable referring to "data" and employing technical vocabulary, find it hard to respond. Mutual trust and communication are difficult to achieve.

Partnerships are also hampered by gaps in information that individual helpers have about the services provided by other helpers and other helping systems. Not only are professionals unaware of the important roles played by lay helpers, but the lay helpers themselves fail to appreciate the scope, magnitude and effect of services that they, themselves, are providing.

This isolation of helping networks is evident on both an intra- and internetwork basis. The Neighborhood and Family Services Project discovered Roman Catholic clergy in neighborhood parishes who were unaware of each other's counseling roles; administrators of closely located mental health clinics who had never met even though they served the same neighborhoods; a lay helper who was totally unaware of another lay helper, living only a few blocks away, who was performing similar services for neighbors.

On the internetwork level, widespread knowledge of each others' actual and potential roles by lay and professional helping networks similarly hampers effective system linkage.

In proposing linkages between community support systems and mental health delivery systems, we are well aware of possible dangers. The temptation to use community support systems to replace public monies in an era of economic scarcity is one such danger. Another is that professionals may inadvertently subvert community support systems by trying to incorporate lay helpers into their agency programs. This can occur when lay helpers become agency volunteers or undertake tasks for the agency on an ad hoc basis. The community helper may then come to be viewed as unpaid staff, not a separate helping entity.

Our experience also indicates that agencies begin to compete to work with community helpers and flood a community with requests for program linkages. Interagency competition may follow.

There is also a danger that, in the enthusiasm for forming partnerships, the process of forming links over time may be circumvented. This sometimes results when agencies require a quick outcome or product such as a new service or program from a partnership. Such circumventions, we believe, will eventually lead to an undermining of community support systems.

Although the dangers are real and the obstacles are formidable, a rational, planned system of linkages is essential. Community helpers are already working with professional mental health and human service providers in many neighborhoods and communities around the United States. What is needed are mechanisms to catalyze the neighborhood potentials and reduce the administrative, fiscal, and legal obstacles that hamper progress. A capacity-building model and a framework of national policy initiatives to help achieve this is proposed in the following section.

A Mental Health Capacity-Building Model: The Empowerment Process

Model Approach

The capacity-building model is developed through a community-empowerment process that is community-directed and agency-linked through which residents become aware of their own strengths, resources, and abilities to shape services to meet neighborhood needs. Central to this process model is the importance of neighborhood. The model utilizes a systems approach based upon the neighborhood as the locus for service and as the basis for preventive and rehabilitative programming. The focus is on the system, rather than on the individual client, because we want to change the interrelated administrative, fiscal, and legal procedures that prevent effective delivery of mental health and human services to residents on the neighborhood level.

Assumptions

The capacity-building model is based on the following basic assumptions that are amply supported in the literature:

1. We live in a pluralistic society. Different groups of people solve problems, face crises, and seek help in various ways because of age, class, race, ethnic, geographic factors, etc. Social class and ethnicity, specifically, are very important variables affecting attitudes toward, and use of services. Yet, class and ethnic differences are often ignored by the service-delivery system, which tends to be designed and operated on a monolithic framework model.

2. Neighborhood and neighborhood attachment are positive resources that can and should be used as a basis for mental health and human service delivery. People need to feel that daily life is being conducted at a manageable scale; in the urban setting, this occurs largely within the neighborhood. Neighborhood has been used as a locus for service for some comprehensive mental health centers, but as little more. There are many strengths and helping resources in communities (friends, neighbors, family, clergy, schools, etc.). Professional services should be designed to strengthen and augment these resources.

3. A sense of competency, self-esteem, and power is extremely important to the well-being of the community. Professional services should be designed to build competency and to build power for the community. This necessitates a radical change in the role of the community and the role of the mental

health and human service professional in the current service system.

4. The community, not agencies, needs to take primary responsibility for its own well-being. We need to rethink the role of professional services vis-à-vis the role of the local neighborhood in providing supports to community members.

5. The mental health system needs to become fully integrated; such integration should involve all service delivery elements. Partnerships are needed among and between the lay and professional helping systems; such partnerships should include the community, private-agency, and governmental sectors.

Overview

   The capacity-building model uses the neighborhod not only as a locus of service but also as:

   a support system and vehicle for the development and strengthening of networks, professional and lay;
   a basis for the development of mental health programming;
   a means of citizen/client involvement; and
   a basis for citizen empowerment in mental health

This view of neighborhood in the provision of mental health helps to overcome obstacles of fragmentation, lack of accessibility, and lack of accountability. It ensures that programs and services will be built upon the unique strengths and resources of particular communities.
   The lay network is defined to include those helpers who provide support services on a voluntary basis to individuals in the community (see Figure 4–1). Lay helpers may have professional training, but the

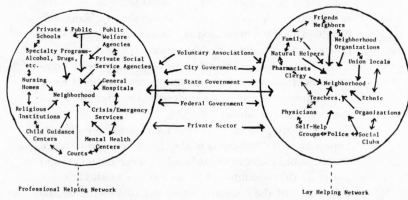

Figure 4–1. Macro System.

helping services they provide are an adjunct, and not a principal part, of their professional training and practice. For example, pharmacists or physicians may provide informal counseling for their customers or patients. The professional network is defined as those individuals that are paid to provide support services to individuals in the community. These support services are provided in an agency or institutional context, usually by professionally trained individuals.

As Figure 4–1 shows, there are actual and potential communication channels and linkages between and among the various helpers, both professional and lay, and to the macro system as well, which represents the larger forces that impact on that relationship. This model represents an ideal. It is not a program model in that it needs to be developed over time and through a series of developmental stages.

Goals

The following are goals of the capacity-building model and a brief description of the issues that need to be addressed in achieving those goals:

Create Community Awareness of Neighborhood Strengths and Needs. Organizationally, the process should work through a local community-based organization or such a group should be developed. This group should have a task force of neighborhood residents directing the effort. The sponsoring organization might be a neighborhood organization, a church or religious group, or ethnic club, etc., depending on the community. By placing the sponsorship and ownership of the process squarely with the community from the beginning, the residents automatically acquire the strength and resources to define for themselves their own needs and resources.

Self-assessment is an extremely important issue. If someone from the mayor's office says that the residents in neighborhood *A* have emotional problems and are in the need of services, then that neighborhood is immediately labelled as a "problem neighborhood," and thereby stigmatized. If, instead, the people in the neighborhood talk with their leaders, doctors, pharmacists, school personnel, human service workers, and their lay helpers, and find out that residents are experiencing a variety of problems, not only have they, themselves, defined the problem, but they reinforce the strengths of the community as well as identifying its problems. Using the traditional clinical analogy: we know that to help someone, we must begin with their presentation of the problem, not ours.

Action research is an indispensable methodological tool for self-assessment. Using action research, community residents, directed by the residents' task force, can gather data and information on help-giving and help-receiving in the neighborhood through collection of "objective" statistical data and through "subjective" interviews with community leaders and helpers. In the course of gathering and analyzing data, issues are clarified and action plans developed.

If the model is to be successful in developing linkages with the professional mental health and human service systems, professionals from a wide variety of service agencies need to be involved. A professional advisory committee (PAC) should be formed. Its member should be persons holding decision-making positions in their agencies so that they can influence an agency to commit resources to needed projects. This group would be advisory to the task force and would meet on an as-needed basis. Individual members will be further involved as members of task force committees formed to develop action plans to meet identified needs.

Strengthen Neighborhood Helping Networks. This part of the process includes developing linkages among natural helpers in the community; between helper and neighborhood leaders; and among neighborhood residents themselves. The planning process for developing programs, in itself, helps to strengthen the neighborhood helping networks. Clergy, natural helpers, and neighborhood leaders can be brought together through workshops, symposia, and other meetings as part of an action research process. They can then be further involved through work on committees of the task force. One of the goals of any specific program intervention, such as a community-directed primary prevention program, would be that it be organized by a formula to strengthen the neighborhood helping networks.

Strengthen the Professional Helping Networks. Professionals should be advisors to a community-directed process led by community residents. This contrasts with the traditional model in which citizens are advisors to a professional process. The PAC process, itself, will help strengthen the often fragmented and uncoordinated professional helping system by bringing professionals who serve a common neighborhood into regular contact with each other. By initially keeping the PAC and task force separate from one another, community residents will have time to develop knowledge and expertise, and the professionals will be able to examine ways in which they can provide increased support to the lay-helping network.

Form Linkages Between the Lay and Professional Helping Networks. As program committees are formed, task force members might invite professionals to work with the committees to contribute their particular expertise. By the time this occurs, the PAC meeting process will have sensitized most of the professionals to the real ability of the community to develop programs that can work. The two systems will then be able to develop a partnersip, fully aware of their differing roles and agendas.

Programs will operationalize the concept of cosponsorship to create broad-based appeal and legitimacy. For instance, a publicity brochure for a series of family communication workshops could list all the churches, agencies, and groups which support the project. A socialization center for former mental patients might be set up in a church and be run by the community with professional consultation and assistance. Not only does such a system decrease the stigma attached to seeking help, it also links services for more effective utilization, extends the resources of the community agencies, and meets needs for community control and agency support.

Form Linkages Between the Lay and Professional Helping Networks and the Macro System.   Once the neighborhood process is well on its way, the community needs to begin to look at the larger forces which impact on the process and represent resources, obstacles, and incentives to institutionalization of the community process. Necessary linkages must take place at many levels so that federal, state, and local programs do not create further obstacles and disincentives to an effective service delivery system for neighborhood residents. Task force and PAC members can put together a data base of information regarding state and local mental health and human service plans; United Way Funding patterns; agency program plans; major pending legislation, etc. They can scout local funding possibilities, and communicate with local foundations, industry, and other funding services. This stage of the process is critical if the accomplishments of the process are to be long-standing.

Models such as the above can be successful only if community support systems are recognized as legitimate service-providers by public policy.

FOOTNOTES

1. There is no clear demarcation between mental health services and human services. Mental health services are currently focused on two groups of people—*the severely ill* who suffer from overpowering depressions, suicidal impulses, loss of contact with reality, major disorders of thought, severe delusions, etc.;

and *the worried well*—who need assistance with the problems, stresses, and crises of everyday life which lead to loneliness, sadness, tensions, and marital discord. Although both groups can benefit from nonpsychiatric assistance, it is clear that the worried well especially are not the exclusive concern of the mental health service system. The worried well can, and should, receive assistance from a wide variety of human service agencies. They can be especially helped by community support systems. Our use of the term mental health pertains principally to the worried well, and also implicitly encompasses human services for this population group.

2. The Neighborhood and Family Services Project is a four-year NIMH-funded research and demonstration effort aimed at strengthening neighborhood and family life by identifying and removing obstacles which prevent community residents from seeking and receiving help. It is a process that focuses on the unique strengths and helping resources of neighborhoods and builds upon these resources to create linkages between community and professional helping networks. This leads to redirection of existing resources and creation of new programs to meet unmet needs. For further information about the project, contact the Washington Public Affairs Center, University of Southern California, 512 10th Street, NW, Washington, D.C. 20004.

REFERENCES

Agranoff, R. Services integration, in Anderson, W. Frieden, B., and Murphy, M., eds. *Managing human services.* Washington, D.C.: International City Management Association, 1977.

Barbarin, O., Mitchell, R., and Hurley, R. Experience of community life: Applying an open-system model of community. Unpublished paper.

Barrabe, P. and Von Mering, O. Ethnic variation in mental stress in families with psychotic children. *Social Problems,* 1953, *1,* 48–53.

Berger, P. and Neuhaus, R. *To empower people: The role of mediating institutions.* Washington, D.C.: American Enterprise Institute for Public Policy Research, 1977.

Breton, R. Institutional completeness of ethnic communities and the personal relations of immigrants. *American Journal of Sociology,* 1964, *70*(2), 193–205.

Caplan, G. *Support systems and community mental health.* New York: Behavioral Publications, 1974.

Caplan, G. and Killilea, M. eds. *Support systems and mutual help.* New York: Grune and Stratton, 1976.

Collins, A. and Pancoast, D. *Natural helping networks: A strategy for prevention.* Washington, D.C.: National Association of Social Workers, 1976.

Dohrenwend, B. P. and Dohrenwend, B. S. *Social status and psychological disorder.* New York: Wiley, 1969.

Dohrenwend, B. P. and Dohrenwend, B. S. *Social status and psychological disorder: Causal inquiry.* New York: Wiley-Interscience, 1976.

Doughton, M. J. *People power.* Bethlehem, Pa.: Media America, 1976.

Fandetti, D. and Gelfand, D. Attitudes toward symptoms and services in the ethnic family and neighborhood. *American Journal of Orthopsychiatry,* 1978, *48*(3), 477.

Giordano, J. *Ethnicity and mental health.* New York: American Jewish Committee, 1973.

Glazer, N. The limits of social policy. *Commentary,* 1971, *52*(3), 51.

Gurin, G., et al. *Americans view their mental health.* New York: Basic Books, 1960.

Hollingshead, A. and Redlich, R. *Social class and mental illness, a community study.* New York: Wiley, 1958.

Hurley, R. *Poverty and mental retardation: A causal relationship.* New York: Random House, 1969.

Langner, T., Herson, J., Green, E., Jameson, J., and Goff, J. Children of the city: Affluence, poverty, and mental health, in Allen, V., ed., *Psychological factors in poverty.* Chicago: Markham, 1970.

Litwak, E. Voluntary associations and neighborhood cohesion. *American Sociological Review,* 1961, *26*(2).

Myers, J. and Bean, L. *A decade later: A follow-up to social class and mental health.* Wiley, 1968.

Naparstek, A. *Policy options for neighborhood empowerment.* Washington, D.C.: National Urban Policy Roundtable, 1976.

Naparstek, A., Spiro, H., et al. *Neighborhood and family services project, first year annual report.* Washington, D.C.: University of Southern California, Washington Public Affairs Center, 1977.

Naparstek, A., Biegel, D., et al. Community analysis data report, Vol. I, first level analysis. *Catalogue of Selected Documents in Psychology,* Manuscript #1964, November, 1979.

Opler, M. *Culture and social psychiatry.* New York: Atherton Press, 1967.

Redlich, R. and Goldsmith, H. 1970 census data used to indicate areas with different potentials for mental health and related problems. NIMH Methodology Reports, Series C, No. 3. *Public Health Service Publication* No. 2171, April, 1971.

Riessman, F., Cowen, J., and Pearl, J. *Mental health of the poor.* New York: Crowell-Collier, 1964.

Sarason, S., et al. *Human services and resource networks.* San Francisco: Jossey-Bass, 1977.

Slater, P. *The pursuit of loneliness: American culture at the breaking point.* Boston: Beacon Press, 1970.

Snyder, J. The use of gatekeepers in crisis management. *Bulletin of Suicidology*, Fall, 1971.

Spiegel, J. Some cultural aspects of transference and counter transference, in Zald, M., ed. *Social welfare institutions*. New York: Wiley, 1965.

Srole, L., et al. *Mental health in the metropolis: the midtown Manhattan study*. New York: McGraw-Hill, 1962.

Warren, D. Neighborhood in urban areas, in Turner, J., ed. *The encyclopedia of social work*. New York: National Association of Social Workers, 1977.

Zborowski, M. *People in pain*. San Francisco: Jossey-Bass, 1964.

Part II

HEALTH-HEALING INTERVENTIONS

Chapter 5

THE PERSONAL HEALTH EXPLORATION

Psychosocial Intervention with Physical Illness

Dennis T. Jaffe, Ph.D.

In this chapter Dennis Jaffe argues effectively that medical symptom-based treatment, intervening within the biological level of the human system, although critical, is limited in its scope. The author presents documented evidence of the psychosocial factors contributing to illness on interpersonal, behavioral, cognitive and emotional levels. A new psychosocial intervention approach to health crisis is described, requiring patients to undertake an active role in their own healing, in collaboration with the physician and a health guide (therapist). With the assistance of his/her health guide, the patient is provided new skills and abilities for coping with his/her health problems.

The Personal Health Exploration is the process which aims to increase the patients' abilities to respond effectively to their life crisis. This process involves three stages; the personal inquiry stage, allowing the guide to intervene psychotherapeutically and educationally with the patient; a self-regulating training stage, a didactic program providing the patient's stress reducing and coping techniques and methods; and a mobilization and transformation stage, an individualized change program where patients are able to modify negative habits and styles of life to more productive and less stressful ones.

ELEMENTS OF A PERSONAL HEALTH EXPLORATION

People come to me for a variety of reasons. They are not recovering from their illness or they have a chronic condition for which they have been told there is no treatment. Others feel that there is more that they could be doing to help themselves get well or stay well, or they intuit that something about their life in general, and its stress level, has led to their current crisis. What they have in common is a desire to understand their illness more fully, and a desire to become more active in overcoming it. I will not accept a person for treatment who is not under a physician's care.

A single woman, age 35, living alone, consulted me when a minor operation for a cervical cyst was not healing after several months. The immediate reason we uncovered was that she felt resentful of her physician, who insisted she return to work before she felt she had healed fully. When she wrote him about her feelings, she healed almost immediately. The next question we explored was why she had the disease at all. Her denial of sexuality, loneliness, the emptiness and lack of meaning in her life all may have decreased her resistance to illness. Slowly, she has begun to modify some of these aspects of her life, within the context of a health support group.

A man who was overweight, diabetic, and hypertensive came to me because he had trouble modifying his diet, and because he wanted to make his life less stressful. Many areas in his life were explored, and he discovered many reasons for his lack of self-care. First, his wife was like a mother to him, continually nagging him to do things differently, leaving him feeling angry and rebellious at her interference with his autonomy. Second, a continual conflict with his business partners, whom he feared confronting, made him dread going to work. Third, a sense of malaise, of having nothing further to look forward to, and of not having done something meaningful with his life, hung over him. Fourth, his marriage and family were routinized, with little emotional or sexual intimacy or satisfaction. Eating was one of his few self-nurturing outlets. Thus, his symptoms seemed to be multidetermined, and a course of individual and couple therapy was begun, leading gradually to increasing control over his symptoms, as well as heightened satisfaction and sense of well-being.

The psychotherapeutic/educational intervention I will discuss for people with physical illness is best labelled a personal health exploration. It consists of a four-to-ten-session course of psychotherapy with the patient (whom I rename the "participant," to reinforce his or her more active role), and at times other family members. The program also includes a four-meeting class in relaxation, stress management, and self-regulation, which includes daily homework (practice with tapes, writing in a journal and personal health workbook, and several experiential/self-reflective exercises). Often, the exploration is followed by participation in a self-help support group, which brings together several people struggling with the crisis or consequences of illness, all trying to initiate major change in their lives and personal styles. This model is based on my experience with a five-day inpatient psychiatric unit (Jaffe, 1975), and on models of personal change which look at psychosocial transition (Parkas, 1971) as necessitating a change of coping style and a remobilization of inner and outer resources for life change (Gould, 1978).

Conceptually, I can make a distinction between three stages or phases in the intervention process, although they overlap and interconnect in practice: (1) personal inquiry, (2) self-regulation training, and (3) mobilization and transformation. Phase 1, the *personal inquiry*, is a mutual exploration, between health guide (therapist) and participant (patient), often including spouse and other family members, into the participant's personal history, significant life events, the meaning and purpose of their life, and the external and internal factors that predisposed, triggered, and maintained illness. The second phase, *self-regulation training*, is an educational experience in self-awareness, body awareness, methods of relaxation, self-healing, stress management, and techniques for achieving a more effective personal health-care system. The final phase, *mobilization and transformation*, includes activation of planned change in life style, behavior, thought processes, and emotional responses which enable the participant to adapt to life more effectively and maintain a higher level of health.uu13No matter how deeply the participant has slipped into the traditional passive, victimized, disconnected patient role, the personal health exploration is a conscious process of reeducation toward the new active, involved, holistic role. The traditional dyad of passive patient, and all-knowing, all-powerful physician becomes transformed in the course of the counseling process into the new, triadic, balanced interrelationship of physician, activated patient, and health guide, working together, each with their particular responsibilities, functions, and roles, to create health. The exploration gives the patient something to do, if possible for hours each day. There is writing in a journal, and scores of exercises and techniques to practice, and a whole life to redefine, if necessary.

In this stage of treatment, the patient/participant is in charge, assessing his needs, learning new skills, and implementing life change. With increasing activity, involvement, and control, this healing relationship also forms a model, and an example, for increased autonomy and self-control in other areas of life. This process reverses some of the negative psychological and interpersonal consequences of the crisis of illness. Instead of feeling more isolated and less in control, the participant learns to experience greater control, to become more aware of his needs and feelings and his ability to meet them, and to share this learning with his family, who in other circumstances might withdraw or find it difficult to relate to him.

I have utilized this type of intervention in several clinical settings. It is the basic mode of service in my private psychosomatic medical clinic, Learning for Health. I have worked with several physicians to incorporate the exploration into their clinical practice, with nurses, social workers, or counselors acting as the health guides. In inpatient and residential settings, the exploration is part of the program of the UCLA Center for Health Enhancement (a 24-day residential program whose goal is to educate people with serious illness, especially heart disease, obesity, and diabetes, to become more active in promoting their health through nutrition, exercise, and stress management), and has been used in several hospitals for people facing surgery or who are critically ill. It is a fairly low-cost program.

Research and assessment of the extent and nature of the effects of the exploration have only just begun. Rosen and Wiens (1979) report that a similar psychological program led to decreased use of medical services in a clinic. However, because the intervention is so global, with so many targets and so many forms, assessment is difficult. It has different effects on different people, and there seem to be few consistencies or commonalities in the responses or effects on people with similar diseases. Pilot research is under way to assess some of the effects of this intervention, and to link them with severity of illness, type of illness, and different personal styles.

Another question that has been asked about this intervention concerns participation. Positive change, critics maintain in response to the research reported by Simonton, Simonton, and Creighton (1978) for their five-day residential program for cancer patients, results from the special, self-selected nature of the people who choose to participate in this very intense, self-reflective process. These patients would have done well anyway, because they already had self-regulated coping mechanisms. If this mode of intervention is to become widespread, then work must be done in learning how to present and facilitate involvement in the treatment process of populations, such as poorer and particularly fearful or externally oriented groups, who would not be expected to elect this type of activity.

While I too have worked largely with a self-selected population, my experience, and that of other health guides, is that with a careful orientation and presentation, a majority of seriously ill people will elect such a program. Although psychosocial exploration cannot be imposed, when the rationale and possible benefits of this experimental program are outlined, many people who would not have requested it welcome the opportunity to bring "themselves" into treatment. Yet, some patients have fears of exploring past events or painful feelings, or difficulty believing that such reflections have any relevance to their health, or are not willing to make any changes in their lives. They may elect not to participate, or, more often, to enter only certain aspects of the process. Many people desire only the self-regulation training component, which they recognize as useful to their health, but do not wish to undertake the inquiry or change phases. The class or workshop format is less threatening. Sometimes, after a few weeks or even months of practice in self-regulation techniques, the person will return to begin counseling. Another common choice is for spouse or family not to participate, for a variety of reasons, ranging from lack of involvement or time, to fear or hostility or indifference to the ill person.

Stage 1: The Personal Inquiry

Motivating.   Despite a frequent readiness for the severely ill to agree to "do anything I can" to promote health, the type of engagement and collaboration demanded in the personal health exploration cannot take place without a period of preparation and orientation by the guide. In order to make an informed choice to enter the process, and then to complete the work at home, in counseling and in classes, a complete explanation of the basic assumptions and expectations of the active patient role must precede the inquiry. In order to complete the exploration, the participant must be highly motivated.

I use reading materials, lectures, and explanation in the initial interview to explain clearly what is expected. I give participants a personal health workbook, which contains articles, explanations, outlines, self-assessment questions for the inquiry phase, and exercises for home practice. Participants are encouraged to read some of the workbook first, and most of them have the time and inclination to do so.

The most important and most difficult theme that needs to be understood is that illness and symptoms might be related to any aspect of one's life, and that the type of reflection and change demanded by the program entails long and hard work, on a daily basis, and willingness to consider major life changes. Often I use a contract, or learning agreement, which explicitly sets forth the responsibilities and expectations of the participant. This orientation process is critical, because the interaction that begins here is the model for all succeeding phases of the process.

History and Systems Review.   I begin the interview by asking about the current physical crisis, or chronic symptom, and in general what was going on in the participant's life in the year or so prior to the onset that might contribute to the stress leading to breakdown. If the symptom is chronic or recurring, I inquire into its patterns, what is going on prior to and at the moment the symptom occurs. The intention is to place the symptom or illness into the broader life context in which it takes place, to begin to discover its meaning and significance.

There are almost always triggering stresses, trauma, or events, not only for major breakdowns, but for the onset of each minor symptom. For example, people with chronic pain such as headache often discover repressed, unexpressed, or unheeded anger, frustration or dislike, or buildup of physical tension, just prior to the pain. Major illnesses relate to losses of job, people in the family (often parents, spouses, or children moving out), or of meaning or pleasure in life. A woman with cancer reported that a few months before she had suffered financial reverses, and began to dread the thought of growing old without adequate financial security, always having to work at her unfulfilling job. She felt she gave up on life before she was diagnosed as having cancer. Sometimes the triggering factor is guilt, perhaps about sexuality. A woman developed a tumor several months after an abortion, another man an ulcer soon after admitting to himself that he was gay. The triggering event very often is an unresolved emotional trauma or life change.

I also inquire into the consequences of the illness, on the person, his sense of himself and the future, and on family and work. I always find some secondary gain which complicates the recovery process; there are always psychosocial benefits to being ill. Illness is often the only allowable way to take a rest or vacation. It becomes clear that illness can be a covert way for a person to compel, nurture, or feel justified in asking for something for themselves. Often, an illness will strike a self-denying, unselfish person who always gives to others—her family, people at work—but can never ask for themelves. I always ask people to define one or more benefits of illness in their lives, and have yet to find a person who cannot define one.

Then I begin a review of social, family, behavioral, cognitive, and emotional systems, to understand what personal dissatisfactions, conflict, self-defeating habits, trauma, past events, or changes might have weakened a person's resistance to illness. The outline I follow is similar to the personal systems review or Ireton and Casseta (1976). My goal is to pinpoint all potential contributors to the current illness and to illuminate the person's customary responses to stress and tension.

Specific dysfunctional responses to stress emerge in this interview. For example, many people suppress all of their needs and responses to stress. A woman with severe gastrointestinal disease reported that she could not express anger or make demands on her family, even though she knew that her frustration increased her gastric secretion to a dangerous level. Many people allow conflicts or difficulties to exist continually without feeling it is possible to resolve them. A man with severe stress symptoms felt that he was completely powerless to have his wife stop interfering in his daily affairs, and checking up on him behind his back. Still others experience a continual cycle of worry or anticipatory or retrospective anxiety—they replay negative situations or imagine negative outcomes, thoughts which have the physiological effect of arousing their stress response in the absence of an environmental threat. In every initial interview, significant patterns of maladaptive response to life stress, and specific events and difficulties, can be related to current symptoms.

After this interview, I ask the participant to take the personal health workbook home, and spend some time each day reflecting on the questions there. They include many of the questions about personal history and psychosocial systems that I have already asked, as well as some short-answer and self-scoring inventories about stress responses and life change. (Most of these questions are included in the Appendix.) In this way they begin to keep a personal journal, and get into the habit of reflecting on their lives and relating their personal worlds to their physical symptoms. The workbook questions focus on all the factors outlined earlier that researchers have suggested relate to host resistance to illness.

Mirroring and Focusing.   As a health guide, rather than a psychotherapist, I adopt a role that is close to the Rogerian (1961) or client-centered style of counseling. My role is to ask important questions, and then to reflect on possible answers offered by the participant. Rarely do I interpret hidden feelings, motivations, or unconscious activities, as I might in longer-term psychotherapy. Continually I mirror back to the participant themes that seem important, trying to help the participant isolate and define that major factors that contributed toward, maintain and triggered illness. My goal is to maximize the participant's control over the process, and to build greater self-awareness and internal sensitivity in the participant. The process then becomes a skill that is internalized and can be used to maintain health in the future and avoid symptoms.

By the second or third session, the participant is able to define the major conflicts, feelings, stress response patterns, and interpersonal factors that relate to his or her illness. It is the participant, not the guide, who determines which factors are important and which areas of life need to change.

Creating Meaning.   What we are doing in the inquiry process is to help the participant to make the initially irrational, random, and unplanned event of illness take on meaning within the person's life. My assumption is that the peculiarly human process of looking at disease not as an intruder or irrational occurrence, but one which is intimately and directly connected with the entire fabric of a person's life, is somewhat relevant to the outcome of treatment. Even the symbolic, personal significance of an illness is taken into account, in the aspect of the inquiry that involves drawing and making mental pictures of one's illness. In her influential book, *Illness as Metaphor*, Sontag (1978) portrays the mythology and social imagery that have grown up around two diseases of society—tuberculosis and cancer—and then she dismisses these as irrelevant and destructive to the medical process of treatment. My experience has been that the personal and social imagery surrounding a symptom is not without truth, and provides important clues to the personal and emotional factors that help to trigger ailments. Usually, the pain and struggle of the body have a parallel-related psychological arena of pain and struggle, often denied or not consciously addressed, which is explored in the inquiry.

Lockhart (1977) and Achterberg and Lawlis (1978) have both looked at the symbolic meaning that people attach to mental imagery of their disease. Achterberg and Lawlis have related patient's mental images of their cancer, and their body's ability to resist (white blood cells) the disease, to the outcome of treatment, much as Klopfer (1957) did a generation earlier, predicting from the symbolic responses to Rorschach inkblots which patients had fast growing tumors. If the inner images contain more vividness, size, color, movement, and potency to the disease image, then the prognosis is poor, if the power lies with the white blood cells, the outcome is better.

I have people draw pictures of their illness, and their body's resources for combating it, and explore with them their inner feelings, expectations, imagery, and symbolic significance they have for their illness and the power of their body in general. If a person cannot picture their illness, picture themselves being healed of it, or picture themselves as well, that usually suggests some inner conflict or resistance to getting well. People's feelings about the nature and meaning of their illness, even if they have no physiological basis, usually relate to important themes in their lives.

One particular theme shows up commonly in relation to imagery of illness. Illness and symptoms often arise in people who have disowned certain feelings, potentialities in themselves, or who lead unbalanced, one-dimensional lives. For example, many men who come to me with heart problems relate them to an absence of love and intimacy in lives which were consumed by career and ambition. A woman with a life-threatening degenerative illness found that the attacks got worse as she completed professional school, in a field that she had chosen to follow in her father's footsteps. The message was that she needed to pick another profession.

I utilize two techniques in this area of the inquiry. First, I have people cultivate body awareness, particularly emotions and sensations that occur at the site of their symptom or disease. Second, I have people create spontaneous mental images concerning their illness, and concerning factors in their life which might contribute to it. I find myself asking people to look into themselves and to simply ask themselves what factors in their life relate to their illness, or need to be changed to promote recovery. I find that these are powerful techniques that are invaluable in this form of exploration (Bresler, 1979; Jaffe, 1980; Jaffe and Bresler, 1980; Segal, 1980).

A word has to be said concerning Sontag's accusation, which has been levelled erroneously at people like myself who wish to connect personal meaning with illnesses, that the use of personal inquiry into factors affecting illness amounts to the addition of one more burden on the sufferer, a dose of "blaming the victim" for his disease. The phrase that has become popular, "taking responsibility for one's illness," seems to have this connotation, that a person has personally, self-destructively, helped to create one's illness.

When I conduct the inquiry, I do not see the participants feel this sense of weight, guilt, or accusation. That is because I very strictly refrain from making interpretive comments, such as "your angry feelings about your wife may have affected your ulcerated stomach." I say to people that it is up to them to make the connections, and that the purpose of the inquiry is to look for current burdens, stress factors, and emotional/interpersonal conflicts that are currently adding to their illness, so that they may be changed. The emphasis clinically is on the present and future, not on regret and past events. To tell patients that they can change their future for the better is not the same as to blame them for what they have neglected in the past.

Family Sharing.   I have stopped considering illness as lying within a single individual. While the breakdown and symptoms are manifest physiologically within one person, the entire life system can have patterns which create and maintain symptoms. This is especially true within families. Minuchin, Rozman, and Baker (1978) have demonstrated that a whole family can have a synchronized biopsychosocial system that leads to breakdown in one member's body. The family, they suggest, has one body. When family patterns are altered, to support greater flexibility and individual autonomy, then the symptoms disappear (Jaffe, 1978).

I have the spouse or family of the ill person come in for one or more interviews, to conduct a version of the inquiry for the whole family. Illness can be a great disorganizer or transformer of family roles. The danger of the illness can increase closeness and caring, or breed isolation. One person's illness makes demands on other family members which might lead to guilt or resentment. It is often important for the whole family to air deep feelings in order for healing to take place.

In one family, where the husband was critically ill, the family conflict involved resentment at the husband who had lost his job and did not attempt to get another. He felt the others' criticism, and the family felt that this related to his breakdown. His illness enabled him to share his own fears and pain, which previously he was denying. In other families the core issues relating to the symptoms have to do with continual conflict in the couple, or a pattern of avoidance or disengagement, or overinvolvement. Either extreme can breed physical expression of the conflicts. For example, in a couple where an alcoholic husband reformed after 20 years, he developed a disabling heart attack which placed him once more as a dependent in his wife's care. Another woman became ill soon after she seriously considered leaving her husband.

There is only space here for a brief description of the richness of this phase of the exploration. Within the space of a few sessions, people in crisis make connections in their life they have never seen before, and explore issues which they had previously denied. The loose structure which suggests areas of inquiry, but allows the participant to determine significance and focus, reinforces the patient's autonomy. What has been most interesting to me in undertaking this process with more than a hundred people is how congruent the inquiry is with common sense assumptions about illness. Thus, although the biomedical model denies individual participation in the creation of illness, or downplays its significance, individuals themselves spontaneously think about these notions when they are ill. Abrams (1966) notes that people with cancer begin by asking the question "Why me?" and looking at personal factors that may have led them to become ill. By guiding the individual, and helping relieve guilt and find constructive outlets for difficult feelings, the process proceeds easily and leaves the participant feeling much better and freer as a result.

Stage 2: Self-Regulation Training

This stage of the health exploration is didactic; it offers training in specific skills of gaining conscious control over physiological functions, especially those having to do with the stress response. This training phase is best conducted in a class or workshop setting, and it can be done without, prior to, or at the same time as the more personal and individualized inquiry process.

Gary Schwartz (1979) suggests that the brain is a complete health-care system, which, during illness, has become dysfunctional. He finds that when a person becomes more aware of his internal functioning, and pays attention to it, the body often becomes in itself self-calibrating, allowing itself to move spontaneously toward greater health. Similarly, the literature regarding relaxation training (or approaches based on meditation, progressive relaxation, autogenic training or self-hypnosis) suggests that a person can learn to activate within the body mechanisms that reverse or prevent the dysfunctional effects of the stress response. Learning to tap these physical capabilities is a universal capacity of the person, which can be activated with a few sessions of training.

Much has been written about self-regulation training (Jaffe, 1980). I have found that a four-to-eight-session class can train people in how to relax their bodies, and activate deep self-regenerative physical capacities. This class demonstrates to people that they can have an effect on their healing process, and on their physical health, and by learning internal self-control, I observe that a person's general sense of personal power and capacity to make a difference in life increases. While the prescription of drugs to deal with stress-related symptoms has zero or negative effect on personal autonomy, self-regulation has a positive effect.

In my training program I teach a graded series of exercises in self-awareness and basic relaxation, and then more specialized techniques of self-healing and stress management. I begin with exercises to help people tune their awareness into their body, which are based on the experiential focusing approach of Gendlin (1978). I find that often physical symptoms get worse because people have not developed the habit of paying attention or following the messages of their bodies. I have people spend the time between their first and second classes stopping several times a day and listening to their bodies.

The next part of the course is relaxation training. The goal is for each participant to learn this basic skill. I use several methods and let participants practice them all and then select the one that works best for them. I begin with progressive deep muscle relaxation (Jacobson, 1962) and then use exercises based on breath meditation (Benson, 1975) and the visceral suggestions of autogenic training (Pelletier, 1977, 1979). When a person does not feel he is learning to relax effectively, I offer biofeedback apparatus to help validate the state of relaxation, or to help learn more effectively. Workshop members keep daily records of their progress in learning relaxation, and are given cassette tapes to help them practice at home. I find that by having a support group and openly discussing the difficulty of making relaxation into a daily habit, adherence to this regime, at least in the form of daily practice during the period of the workshop, can be achieved.

After the basics of attaining a state of deep psychophysiological relaxation have been achieved, then specific exercises are added for particular difficulties. I teach the use of visual imagery to plant suggestions for the body to heal more quickly for those with particular physical symptoms, following the imagery methods described by the Simontons (1978) for cancer patients, and Bresler (1979) with pain patients. I teach people that they can augment or speed up the natural healing processes and the medications of their medical treatment, by using these varieties of inner suggestions.

Another training exercise in the workshop has to do with the use of visual imagery to modify psychophysical responses to stressful situations. People learn to remember or anticipate potential stressful situations, and then practice, within their mind, while relaxed, new responses. Slowly, people learn that they can have some effect on their emotional and habitual patterns of response to life situations. By the end of the workshop each participant will have the customary belief that the body is an autonomous entity, incapable of conscious or willful control, firmly undermined. In its place, most participants have an experiential awareness that they can know how their body feels and what it needs, and can actively manage their psychophysical responses to life stress, and enhance their ability to heal whatever ailments they have developed. For most, the training workshop is a powerful experience, building self-esteem as well as teaching self-management practices that can be used for the rest of their lives.

Courses such as this, with or without the addition of the other aspects of the self-exploration process, are becoming increasingly common in clinics and health settings. The skills that are learned are critical for preventing illness and maintaining health. However, I feel that the specific skills often cannot be applied without the personal exploration and alleviation of personal conflicts and obstacles to health. But a workshop/course like this is a cornerstone of a psychosocial intervention to enhance health, and psychosomatic treatment cannot proceed without it.

Stage 3: Mobilization and Transformation

There are two treatment plans which make up a comprehensive health program. One is the physician's treatment program, the other is the personal health plan which is implemented by the patient. After the personal inquiry and a period of self-regulation training, the individuals in health crisis, and usually their entire family, must create their own personal change program for attaining maximum health. This has been termed a positive wellness program by John Travis, the physician who founded the Wellness Resource Center.

An active program to mobilize new coping skills to respond more effectively to the demands of life which may (or may not) have led to the particular breakdown of illness. In this stage of a health program, a person learns to actively modify negative habits, response patterns or styles of life. For example, a person with heart disease who exhibits the time-dominated, hard-driving, easily frustrated Type-A behavior pattern will need to modify some of these qualities by modifying, for example, the work schedule, learning to relax for short breaks during work, giving up control over projects to peers and subordinates, and practicing techniques of active listening. A person who continually feels helpless and hopeless, or who continually gets anxious by expecting the worst, will have to learn to modify these internal dialogues or assumptions about life, because they threaten future health and recovery from illness.

Each person must develop a change program, after careful consideration of how he individually experiences stress, and the nature of his particular symptoms. The health program usually involves some important changes in central areas of life. For purposes of developing awareness of the spheres of life which a person can change, I suggest the following levels:

1. Environmental changes: Change in social involvements, work, living place, or anything else about the people and places that surround one. One's environment has much to do with how one feels and what one reacts to.

2. Behavioral change: A person can change his behavior in relation to his family, his personal relationships, work, and everyday behavior. People often need to change their food or exercise behavior, or the way they interact with people around them. While it is difficult to change other people, it is often most practical to change one's response to others, which in turn affects their response to us.

3. Change in mental patterns: Worries are anticipated negative events, or replays of past stressful events, which activate our physical stress response even though they are simply thoughts. We often tell ourselves negative things about our potential, our expectations, or our abilities, and in many other ways create internally messages and assumptions about our life which help to create stress and pain. Beliefs, mental patterns, and negative thoughts can be modified using mental imagery, relaxation, self-hypnosis, and psychotherapy.

4. Change in physical responses: Our physical responses to life events can be modified by daily use and practice in psycho-

physiological self-regulation. Using self-regulation can help overcome the negative effects of painful emotional states, and overcome excessive stress when it occurs within the body. However, constrained people are in other areas of their lives, they can always modify their physiological responses to life events.

When people look at their life stress, and the personal dilemmas and painful past and present situations which might lead to their illness or symptoms, the purpose is to find out what things have to be modified in the present to create health or recovery from illness in the future. Each person who undertakes a personal health exploration eventually makes some determinations of factors that influence the illness, and then takes steps to modify those factors. In that way, the person is conservatively taking care of even factors that might just possibly lead to illness. When one's life and health lie in the balance, this sort of excessive caution can be justified.

The change program each person undertakes at this point in the process is different. People who are in life crisis often work through the effects of their life change or crisis emotionally, using conventional psychotherapeutic techniques, and sometimes find that their symptoms decrease or even vanish. Others, whose illness grew up over time due to dysfunctional overreaction or misplaced reaction to stressful situations, learn to modify their responses and behavior.

The shock and pain of breakdown, and the inactive, reflective time that illness offers, both help participants in the personal exploration to consider areas of change and programs which are quite drastic. As can be seen from the examples below, many of these changes, whether or not they affect physical health or recovery, are beneficial in improving the quality of a person's life.

Many people create a health program to alter their life's direction. Since illness demands a decrease in work activity for many, participants often commit themselves to a new area of life. For example, in a group of postbypass surgery men, most of whom had active physical careers, the three men who made the best postoperative adjustment were those who used hobbies or reeducation to form their new work identities. The others remained depressed, largely sitting in front of the television. Several others find that one meaning they derive from their illness is that they do not like their careers and desire either to deemphasize their work life in favor of family activity or to change or modify careers. Many people discover in their reflections that their lives lack joy or pleasure, and that their breakdown reflects an inner depression and giving up. Many times, people connect basic identity issues or the meaning of their lives to their breakdowns.

Another group commit themselves to making changes in their responses to stress, the degree of conflict, anxiety or emotional pain they regularly experience, or to modify a painful, stressful, or conflicted situation they have endured for years. For many ill men and women, the stressful situation they elect to change is their marriages. The marital patterns of continual resentment for intrusion, tyrannical power, or not giving one what one wants, or not being understood, all might be explored under the impetus of illness. Traditional methods of couple or family therapy, cognitive behavior modification, and psychotherapy might be elected at this point.

At this stage of the exploration process, a small group of people with similar illnesses, or who are making changes in their lives, is very important. Self-help groups have a long history as adjuncts or alternatives to psychotherapy, and to help people with the coping process with physical illness (Katz and Bender, 1976; Hurwitz, 1976). What I would suggest is that these benefits of self-help groups might also affect positively the outcome of treatment, although this has not been studied. At the end of the personal health exploration, the people who wish to undertake major life change in restructuring their environments, modifying behavior, altering mental or psychophysiological responses, or changing relationships, are most often invited to join health self-help support groups. They continue for several weeks, to a year or more.

Illness then, is not different from any other sign or symptom of human distress. For the past century, we have assumed that physical ailments were somehow different from and unconnected to other forms of distress, and that therefore, people could be restored to health without any involvement or participation on their part. At the same time, however, elaborate self-participatory processes were developed for alleviation of human psychological distress, to take their place alongside psychosocial healing rituals which existed in all cultures at all periods of history. Now, at a time when medicine is finding the task of responding to the many chronic, vague, nonspecific, degenerative, stress-related illnesses which have no specific physical cause, quite difficult, we need to bring the person back into the treatment process. As they once had been, the whole life of the ill person has to become part of the treatment process.

What this involves is not the rejection of any of the benefits that technological medicine has brought to healing, but rather the addition of psychosocial intervention to the treatment team, and the redefinition of the patient role to a more active, involved, participatory stance. Once more we discover what has always been known, that disease is not a random, irrational occurrence, but is quite often the result of a life that is not lived well. I find, the more I work with illness, that living well is also living in health. Bringing people back to their optimal level of physical health means helping them to live well in a total human sense. The factors that produce human health seem to parallel the factors that create personal well-being.

In summary, the personal health exploration is a model of the clinical activities that might be included within a program of comprehensive, biopsychosocial medical treatment program. My experience is that participation in such a process immeasurably aids patient quality of life, and positive coping mechanisms. Whether such an intervention has a clear, measurable effect on the effectiveness or speed of recovery from disease remains to be studied. Whatever the eventual answer to this question, today, in many medical settings, in the clinical practice of many different health care professionals (nurses, social workers, psychologists, psychiatrists, health educators), the activities that I have written about are increasingly common.

REFERENCES

Abrams, R. D. The patient with cancer—his changing patterns of communication. *New England Journal of Medicine*, 1966, *274*, 317.

Achterberg, J. and Lawliss, F. *Imagery of cancer*. Champaign, Ill.: Institute for Personality and Ability Testing, 1978.

Antonovsky, A. *Health, stress and coping*. San Francisco: Jossey-Bass, 1979.

Bakan, D. *Disease, pain and sacrifice*. Boston: Beacon, 1968.

Beecher, H. K. The powerful placebo. *JAMA*, 1975, *137*.

Benson, H. *The relaxation response*. New York: Morrow, 1975.

Berkman, L. F. Psychological factors, host resistance and mortality. *American Journal of Epidemiology*, in press.

Bowers, K. S. and Kelly, P. Stress, disease, psychotherapy and hypnosis. *Journal of Abnormal Psychology*, 1979, *88*, 5.

Bresler, D. with Trubo, R. *Free yourself from pain*. New York: Simon and Schuster, 1979.

Breslow, L. and Belloc, N. B. The relation of physical health status and health practices. *Preventive Medicine*, 1972, 1, August.

Cannon, W. *The wisdom of the body*. New York: Norton, 1939.

Cantor, R. C. *And a time to live*. New York: Harper & Row, 1980.

Cohen, F. Personality, stress and the development of physical illness, in Stone, G. G., Cohen, F., and Adler, N. E., eds. *Health psychology*. San Francisco; Jossey-Bass, 1979.

Cousins, N. *Anatomy of an illness*. New York: Norton, 1979.

DiMatteo, M. R. and Friedman, H. S. Health care as an interpersonal process. *Journal of Social Issues*, 1979, *35*, 1.

Dohrenwend, B. S. and Dohrenwend, B. P., eds. *Stressful life events*. New York: Wiley, 1974.

Dubos, R. *The mirage of health*. New York: Harper & Row, 1971.

Engel, G. L. The biopsychosocial model and the education of health professionals. *General Hospital Psychiatry*, 1979.

Engel, G. L. A life setting conducive to illness: The giving up–given up complex. *Bulletin of the Menninger Clinic*, 1968, *32*.

Engel, G. L. and Schmale, A. H. Psychoanalytic theory of somatic disorder. *Journal of the American Psychoanalytic Association*, 1967, *15*, 344–365.

Ferguson, T. *Medical self-care*. New York: Summit, 1980.

Frank, J. The faith that heals. *Johns Hopkins Medical Journal*, 1975, *137*.

Gendlin, E. *Focussing*. New York: 1978.

Gould, R. *Transformations*. New York: Simon and Schuster, 1978.

Guttmacher, S. Whole in body, mind and spirit: Holistic health and the limits of medicine. *Hasting Center Report*, 1979, April.

Healthy people. Report of the U.S. Surgeon General, 1979.

Hinkle, L. E., Christenson, W. N., Kane, F. D., Ostfeld, A. M., Thetford, W. N., and Wolff, H. G. An investigation of the relation between life experience, personality characteristics, and general susceptability to illness. *Psychosomatic Medicine*, 1958, *20*.

Hurvitz, N. Origins of peer self-help psychotherapy movement. *Journal of Applied Behavioral Science*, 1976, *12*, 3.

Hutschneker, A. A. *The will to live*. New York: Cornerstone, 1974.

Ireton, H. R. and Cassatta, D. A. A psychological systems review. *Journal of Family Practice*, 1976, *3*, 2.

Jacobson, E. *You must relax*. New York: McGraw-Hill, 1962.

Jaffe, D. T. *Healing from within*. New York: Knopf, 1980.

Jaffe, D. T. The organization of treatment on a short-term psychiatric ward. *Psychiatry*, 1975, *38*, February, 23–38.

Jaffe, D. T. The role of family therapy in treating physical illness. *Hospital and Community Psychiatry*, 1978, *29*, 3, March.

Jaffe, D. T. and Bresler, D. Therapeutic mental imagery: Healing through the mind's eye, in Shorr and Kanella, eds. *Mental Imagery*. New York: Plenum, 1980.

Jenkins, C. D. Social and epidemiologic factors in psychosomatic disease. *Psychiatric Annals*, 1972, *2*, 8–19.

Katz, A. and Bender E., eds. *The strength in us: Self-help groups and the modern world*. New York: Viewpoints, 1976.

Kiely, W. F. Coping with severe illness. *Advances in Psychosomatic Medicine*, 1972, *8*.

Klopfer, B. Psychological variables in human cancer. *Journal of Projective Testing*, 1957, *21*.

Knowles, J., ed. *Doing better and feeling worse: Health care in the United States*. New York: Norton, 1978.

Kroger, W. S. *Clinical and experimental hypnosis*, second edition. Philadelphia: Lippincott, 1977.

LeShan, L. *You can fight for your life.* New York: M. Evans, 1977.

LeShan, L. and Worthington, R. E. Some recurrent life history patterns observed in patients with malignant disease. *Journal of Nervous and Mental Disease,* 1956, *124,* 460–465.

Lazarus, R. S. *Psychological stress and the coping process.* New York: McGraw-Hill, 1966.

MacLean, P. D. Psychosomatic disease and the visceral brain. *Psychosomatic Medicine,* 1949, *11,* 338–351.

Mathews, K. A. et al. Competitive drive, Pattern A, and coronary heart disease. *Journal of Chronic Diseases,* 1977, *30.*

Minuchin, S., Rosman, B., and Baker, L. *Psychosomatic families.* Cambridge: Harvard University Press, 1978.

Nuckolls, K. B., Cassel, J., and Kaplan, B. H. Psychosocial assets, life crisis and the prognosis of pregnancy. *American Journal of Epidemiology,* 1972, *95.*

Parkes, C. M. Psycho-social transitions: A field for study. *Social Science and Medicine,* 1971, *5.*

Paul, N. The use of empathy in the resolution of grief, in Allman, L. R. and Jaffe, D. T., eds. *Readings in adult psychology.* New York: Harper & Row, 1977.

Pelletier, K. R. *Mind as healer, mind as slayer.* New York: Delacort, 1977.

Pelletier, K. R. *Holistic medicine.* New York: Delacort, 1979.

Porritt, D. Social support in crisis: Quantity or quality? *Social Science and Medicine,* 1979, *13A.*

Rodin, J. and Janis, I. L. The social power of health-care practitioners as agents of change. *Journal of Social Issues,* 1979, *35,* 1.

Rogers, C. *On becoming a person.* Boston: Houghton-Mifflin, 1961.

Rosen, J. C. and Wiens, A. N. Changes in medical problems and use of medical services following psychological intervention. *American Psychologist,* 1979, *34,* 5.

Rosenman, R. and Friedman, M. *Type A behavior and your heart.* New York: Knopf, 1974.

Schmale, A. H. Giving up as a final common pathway to changes in health, in Lipowski, Z. J., ed. *Psychosocial Aspects of Physical Illness,* Vol. 8. New York-Basel: Karger, 1972.

Schwartz, G. The brain as a health care system, in Stone, G. C., Cohen, F., and Adler, N. E., eds. *Health psychology.* San Francisco: Jossey-Bass, 1979.

Seligman, M. *Helplessness.* San Francisco: Freeman, 1975.

Selye, H. *The stress of life,* second edition. New York: McGraw-Hill, 1956.

Simonton, O. C., Simonton, S., and Creighton, J. *Getting well again.* Los Angeles: Tarcher, 1978.

Sontag, S. *Illness as metaphor.* New York: Ferrar, Strauss, and Giroux, 1978.

Stephens, J. P. and Henry, J. *Health, stress and the social environment.* New York: Springer Verlag, 1977.

Wolff, H. A concept of disease in man. *Psychosomatic Medicine,* 1962, *24,* 1.

Chapter 6

THERAPEUTIC FAMILY REUNIONS AS A MODERN TRIBAL HEALING

Harold Wise, M.D.

The relationship of the individual, the family, and extended family to social, emotional, and physical stresses and diseases is aptly demonstrated by Harold Wise's use of therapeutic family reunions. His background in internal medicine, enriched by psychotherapy training, has influenced his work in family systems, tribal medicine with its traditions, the healing process and the altered states of healers. He describes six phases of the therapeutic family reunion along with vignettes from three different reunions. The delicate balance between emotional and physical disease and health remains in the foreground throughout.

ORIGIN OF FAMILY REUNIONS

The development of therapeutic family reunions evolved from my work in three different areas: The family as a system, as viewed by both medicine and psychiatry; tribal medicine and its traditions; and the healing process and the altered states of healers.

The Family as a System

In the field of family medicine, which views the family as client, there were several projects which were pivotal for me in my research.

One of these was the Peckham experiment, done in London in 1926, in which the staff would feed back their medical data to the client families in a group meeting. Thus, there was mutual participation in the process of planning for medical care. Another important project was The Family Health Maintenance Demonstration, directed by Dr. George Silver in New York City, in which a health team cared for 150 families in a group medical practice. These families had been randomly selected and matched with controls; the experiment ran from 1952 to 1958. Finally, there is the project I founded in 1964, which is still actively growing, the Dr. Martin Luther King, Jr., Health Center, organized to serve, through health teams, some 12,000 families in the Morrisania section of the southeast Bronx.

In each of these experiments, we looked particularly at compliance with the health care plan developed by the professional staff for the families. Those families which had met with the staff discussed medical and psychological findings, and together with the staff agreed on a plan, and carried out their health care plan 90 percent of the time. I agreed with George Silver that the health care conferences with the entire family present was the most useful encounter with the family, more valuable than any other preventive care strategy.

I will mention the family therapy movement only briefly, because I assume you are familiar with its history, and some of the theoretical work developed by Sullivan, Jackson, Bowen, Whitaker, and Ackerman. A pivotal person in my studies was Michael Balint, the psychoanalyst who brought to the attention of the medical community that individual dysfunction—frequently in a child—may be a presenting complaint of dysfunction in the entire family system.

Tribal Medicine

The second area of study relevant to the family reunion is one of the oldest known forms of healing, the family meeting of tribal medicine. During times of illness, the Kahuna healers of Hawaii, or the tribal elders, call the whole clan together in a ritual called "ho'o, pono, pono." Each person in the clan must express any ill feelings he has to the sick person and must forgive him. The sick person must do the same. Then each person must do the same with everyone else in the tribe. The grudges against one another must be completely forgiven before the healer will work directly on the sick person.

More preindustrial groups had a sense of the importance of the tribe as a whole and would use this kind of meeting for dealing with the illness of one of its members. The American Navajo and the Sioux are groups still practicing this system. The most useful instruction I have had in tribal medicine came from anthropologists Richard Lee (1979) and Richard Katz (1968) and their colleagues, who have worked for the last ten years with the Kung bushmen in Africa's Kalihari. The bushmen probably have the world's oldest living culture and live even now as hunters and gatherers, the way that mankind has lived for 99 percent of its existence.

All the adults of the Kung go through rituals to become healers, although only half complete the process successfully. The role of the healer is given great prestige and is carried out in addition to expected work activities. And although Western medicine is available and used occasionally, bushmen medicine is the most popular form of treatment for both the bushmen and the surrounding tribes.

From Lee's work, I learned that at midlife, the bushmen go through a change and ritual which allows them to pass through a death experience, reaching the "other side"—a state we would probably call another level of consciousness or an unconscious state. This state of bliss they call "Kia." Reaching this state is a very painful process, since the initiate is consumed with fiery energy called "n'um," which is characterized by severe abdominal or chest pain. If the initiate falters, the dance step of the ritual is speeded up, and he is assisted by two more seasoned healers on either side of him. In their language, the pain disappears, the initiate's heart "opens up," the eyes become shiny and clear and the initiate can now deal in two worlds, two levels of consciousness.

Lee made a transcript of the singing during the healing ritual, which he recorded in the early 1970s. What at the time was thought to be incoherent mumblings, on more careful analysis proved to be an exploration by the healer of the sick person's living family system, and the ancestors of the patient who had passed over the "other side."

In Lee's transcript, all the kin, living and dead, are addressed by the healer in the healing ceremony. The healer addresses the sick man's mother, now four years dead:

> Mother, mother. Help your son. Help him. You are angry with him. He was not more caring for you when you were sick and dying. And you love him. You long to bring him to the other side with you. But mother, life is short. Give him this brief time. Let him live. He will join you soon enough. And you, uncle. What are you doing waiting here? You have been dead for seventeen years. I know you love your nephew, but leave him alone. Give him more time in life. Get on your way.

What is important to note is that the whole network of the sick man—both living friends and relatives and the ancestors on the other side—are mobilized for the sick man's recovery. The struggle over the sick man is presented as a tug of war between two loving systems: the sick person's family and friends who want him alive, and those on the other side, equally loving, who want to bring him over with them. The healer, comfortable in both realities, negotiates for life, but understands the pull to the other side is too strong if the man dies. In addressing the dead parents, what I acknowledged is the universal guilt we all feel that we have not done enough for our parents, or other family members who have died while they were alive.

In this country, using approaches derived from family therapy and from tribal medicine, Ross Speck developed a method he called Network Therapy. His early work with Attneave (Speck and Attneave, 1973) and his later work with Rueveni and Joan Speck (Speck and Rueveni, 1977) describes the network process. Speck would assemble the family and friends of the identified patient in the living room of the family home. He would begin the meeting with some kind of dance and song appropriate to the culture of the group he was dealing with. The ground rules included bringing all the family secrets into the open. The rhythm of the meetings tended to follow similar patterns. First there was exuberance that the whole family had assembled. Then there would be a rapid repolarization of alliances in the family. The meeting would come to a stalemate with frustration and despair. Then there was a struggle to build up momentum, followed by a successful breakthrough (or a failure) in resolving the emotional crisis that had brought the family together. The meetings lasted for a long evening, and were often repeated over several weeks. Critical to the success of the process was Speck's development of a network of family and friends to continue meeting around the problem in the intervals between the meetings with the larger family. Speck found that there were usually many overlooked resources in the patient's family and friendship network. For example, the patient might move out of the emotionally charged atmosphere of her immediate family into the emotionally cooler household of an aunt or cousin.

Rueveni (1979) focused on mobilizing the network support for families in crisis. His intervention approaches are reported to be productive in resolving crisis with depressed, suicidal, and psychotic family members. While, of course, the family tended to focus first on the problems of the ailing member, invariably other problems related to the family as a whole were dealt with once one sensed that the atmosphere was supportive.

Healers and the Healing Process

Lawrence LeShan (1969a,b) developed a theory that there were two kinds of healing, which he and colleague Alida Sherman demonstrated. The first kind of healing which LeShan considers minor, involves the theory of energy passing from healer to the person to be healed, the "healee"; this frequently involves minor symptomatic relief. The more important kind of healing, which LeShan finds significant, is the kind in which healer and healee move—both of them—into a shared altered state of consciousness. Here the healer does not try to "cure" the "healee," but rather is "at one with the 'healee'." There is total empathy between the two. Thus, in a certain percentage of cases in this altered state, a healing occurs, dramatic in temporal sequence, but always following basic physiological laws. Every successful healer I have met can enter this shared reality with the "healee," and many in addition work with direct body contact, using the notion of transference of energy as well.

The importance of this shared, altered reality—which Hippocrates called "The Moment Occasio" and Freud called "The Oceanic State"—is that it is the same kind of shared reality I have witnessed in the therapeutic family reunion. As in the bushmen ritual, the entire blood-related family and many of the close kin by marriage enter into a shared, altered state—a state I call the family unconscious. And like Freud's unconscious in individual behavior, the family unconscious is the prime determinant of the emotional life of the members of the family system.

The Family Reunion—Some Vignettes

There are three family reunions that I will draw on to illustrate what happens in such a process. All three reunions were run in marathon meetings of extended families. Although the circumstances for each were quite different, the three families experienced a similar process.

The first family, the Wallachs, came together around the disease—a brain tumor—in their elder daughter, Janet. Janet's uncle, who knew of my work, called to tell me that his niece was in coma, terminally ill with a brain tumor. The girl's mother—his sister—as well as Janet's sister, Kay, younger by ten months, were suffering so much that he felt that both would not survive the ordeal. He asked if anything could be done. That night I met with the uncle, the mother, father, and younger sister, Kay, as well as with Janet's fiancé, while Janet herself lay in a coma in her hospital bed. The meeting continued for an entire evening.

As the story emerged, we tapped into a reservoir of previously unexpected anger centering on the father's history of alcoholism and the mother's greater concern for her business than for the family. These matters came up as the Wallachs described the history of Janet's illness. One week prior to Janet's 18th birthday, which was also the day she was to be married, the mother took Janet for a definitive medical workup for a lifetime history of migraine headaches, which became worse as the wedding approached. The neurologist in Westchester, where the Wallachs lived, did a very careful workup for migraine, and, surprisingly, carried out arteriography—a test which proved normal. Nonetheless, the headaches grew worse, and the wedding was postponed. The neurologist, responding to the alarm in the family, referred Janet to a senior neurosurgeon in New York, who repeated the tests and added a myelogram. This time the neurosurgeon found a lesion in the spinal cord which, on surgery, proved to be a benign ependymoma.

Soon after surgery, the migraines returned. The wedding was cancelled. The family took Janet to another leading neurosurgeon. Since the pathological specimens at the first hospital had been lost, examinations were repeated, and this time, on encephalogram, the radiologists thought there was a tumor in the posterior fossa of the brain. At this point, brain surgery was performed. The diagnosis of benign ependymoma was changed to meningeal gliomatosis with seeding to the spinal cord. The tumor was removed and a bypass inserted. The area was infused locally with cytoxin. Janet's condition began to deteriorate, and she soon went into coma. The resident put her on massive doses of steroids. Her condition worsened, and the staff (several of whom later confirmed the patient's medical history) gave her only a few days to live.

As the Wallachs' story emerged, the father finally exploded in anger against his wife. "There was nothing wrong with Janet," he said to his wife "until you took her to the doctors." While both the mother and father were expressing their anger, the younger sister, Kay, remained silent. There were many indications, however, of a competitive relationship with her more beautiful, older sister who, especially while dying, took center stage. With the martyrdom that usually follows an untimely death, Janet would no doubt continue to take center stage after her death. I sensed that Kay's guilt and anger were paralyzing her. I felt that something had to be changed for her, for otherwise her guilt would grow after Janet's death. As a result, in my strategy I used the younger Kay as my assistant in the healing process.

Because of Janet's terminal condition, it seemed impossible to summon the total extended family to the bedside in the next day or two. I suggested that we try something that I had learned from my study of healing systems, particularly in tribal medicine: A family meditation was suggested in which Janet would be visualized in the center with the immediate family in a circle around her. The mother was enthusiastic. Although the father was skeptical, he agreed to go along with the meditation, and indeed, the Wallachs all later reported feeling a tremendous love flooding Janet and the whole family system.

Before anything could even be arranged with the larger family system, the next day after the meditation Janet came out of coma. This gave the immediate family even greater impetus to connect with the entire family. Two days later the immediate family, along with the uncle and fiancé, met at Janet's bedside. They had synchronized times with the 60-member extended family, who had all set aside this hour to participate in the meditation. At this time, I also spoke to the medical and nursing staff involved in Janet's care, for I knew that if they continued to deal with their patient as if she were terminally ill, there would be no hope of a reversal. I was surprised at the openness of the staff, several of whom agreed to join the Wallachs in the meditation.

The scene at the bedside was very moving. Janet, well under ninety pounds, her head shaved from recent neurosurgery and her face bloated from the steroids, was trying to smile at those around her. The immediate family was at the bedside, with the uncle, the house staff, and nursing staff, and me behind them. The meditation began. Finally the parents could endure it no longer. They moved over to the bed, joined by Kay, and all three wept together, while holding frail Janet in their arms. They joined in this way for half an hour.

It is rare to see this kind of contact at the bedside of a dying person. But here was an open and profound expression of love. I felt that even if nothing more happened, this event had been worth all the energy involved in mobilizing the extended family. The next day Janet's spinal fluid pressure was normal. She was sitting up and taking light foods. There was a debate between the neurologists and neurosurgeons as to whether to do a radium implant. The decision for surgery prevailed, and Janet recovered rapidly; she was discharged from the hospital several weeks later.

The second family, the Alberts, was brought to my attention by a physician who was cousin to a 17-year-old girl named Carla. His call was urgent. The girl was in the intensive care unit of a hospital in Long Island for crushing chest pain. Although she had endured hours of acute pain, and a detailed workup—including EKSs, lab work, and X-rays—showed nothing, the pain and tachycardia continued despite the administration of analgesics, sedation, and cardiac blocking agents. After further tests, nothing else was found. Carla's cousin was a cardiologist, and her uncle a surgeon, and both felt there was an emotional upheaval going on in Carla. She was discharged from the hospital still in pain.

Attempting to get some background information on the Albert family, I learned from the cardiologist that there was a strong history of heart disease on Carla's father's side; and on her mother's side, numerous difficulties. The mother's therapist had been working with both the mother and father for the past year, and with the nuclear family of mother, father, older son, and Carla and her twin brother for several weeks before Carla was hospitalized.

The first battle the therapist must fight is the battle for structure, and this evolved over the issue that the mother and father did not want Carla's grandparents present. I insisted that all three living grandparents attend, as well as all the uncles, aunts, and cousins that could be mobilized in the New York area. The negotiation went on for two days. The father did not want to bring his father—Carla's grandfather—because he had a serious heart condition. I said that I would bring an EKG and a resuscitation cart, and have oxygen on hand and an ambulance on call. The mother said she knew the grandfather would not come. I said then that neither would I. In addition, I insisted that the therapist who had been working with the family be present at the meeting. What I was doing was building up the system, for I sensed that the nuclear family was in too much trouble to make a change by itself, and I needed the support and stability of a larger system if real change and improvement were to occur. Over the telephone, I learned that the parents of Carla were about to see their home become an empty nest, for both Carla and her twin brother were about to join their older brother in an out-of-state college. At the same time the father, who had retired in his early fifties from a demanding business, was now spending a great deal of his time moping around the house.

After numerous phone calls from many members of the family, two days later, 17 members of the extended family—grandfather and the mother's therapist included—met with me in marathon from Friday night until Sunday night. I found the presence of the mother's therapist an invaluable resource to the family and to me. I will return to the Albert family later in the chapter.

The third family was my own family. My younger brother, David, also a therapist, was the brainchild and sparkplug for our therapeutic family reunion, which occurred in August of 1975 when 30 members of my extended family met in marathon with family therapist Carl Whitaker for a three and a half day marathon. We met to see if we could do something about an increasing pattern of cancer developing in the younger members of the family. We were also concerned with the subsequent breakup of the family that had resulted.

THE PHASES OF THE THERAPEUTIC FAMILY REUNION

I would like to outline the steps involved in the family reunion.

1. The Incision: Expression of Anger

There is no better way to describe the first steps of the meeting than as a surgical incision. "Pseudo-mutual" families, such as the Alberts, Carla's family, can find little to be angry about. After 12 hours, all we had gotten to was the fact that one family unit had insulted another family unit by bringing their maid to dinner, wanting her to sit at the table with them. But the anger has to be expressed; it is like dammed-up pus. For, as one member of Carla's family said, "There is so much anger held in here, there is no space to breathe." Carla sat in her chair, mute, holding her chest in pain while her family held this anger in. When this stage comes to a head, so much anger is expressed that you can sense that the air has begun to clear. In Carla's case, as things came slowly out into the open, she brightened up and her pain gradually left her. As mystification and triangulation reappeared, so did her pain and pallor.

In my own family, there was a legacy of anger going back all the way to the 1920s. Particularly painful was the anger expressed by those of the family who had survived Auschwitz and who believed the family in Canada and the United States did not do all they could (before World War II) to save them.

2. Resolution of Unresolved Grief: Acceptance of Guilt

In Carla's family, there was much talk about an uncle who had died at an early age. This family role is what I have come to call the "Lamed Vovnik"[1] of the family, the legend being that there are only 36 righteous people in the world, "Lamed" and "Vov" adding up numerically to 36 in Hebrew. In the Albert family, as in many other families I have seen, the Lamed Vovnik is a saintlike, sacrificial figure who remains a symbol and is never allowed to be a full human being with human frailty to balance the saintly qualities. It appeared to me that Carla had taken on the role of Lamed Vovnik in her family, following in her late uncle's footsteps. In my own family, my grandfather, after whom I was named, had the role, then my uncle, then my mother— with all three dying young. I had inherited the role then, and prior to the family reunion had been doing everything I could to get out of it. And at the reunion itself, my young cousin, Michael, seemed to be taking on the role.

The Lamed Vovnik becomes apparent in the second stage of the reunion, when there is mourning for those members of the family whose deaths have been inadequately mourned. Even though the deaths may have taken place many years before, the grief remains in the system.

Along with the grief is the guilt that the family carries about the Lamed Vovnik and his or her attempts to become a person and not remain a symbol. Usually, when this happens, the family withdraws from the Lamed Vovnik, and like Jesus, the Lamed Vovnik sacrifices himself to save the family.

In my own family reunion, we mourned the death of my mother, who had been the central connecting person for my immediate family as well as for the extended family. The mourning bore a striking resemblance to a passage I remembered from Joyce's Ulysses:

> The ghost of Stephen's dead mother has appeared to him.
> *The Mother*
> (With a subtle smile of death's madness) I was once the beautiful May Goulding. I am dead.
> *Stephen*
> (Horror struck) Who are you? What bogeyman's trick is this?
> *The Mother*
> (Comes nearer, breathing upon him softly her breath of wetted ashes) All must go through it, Stephen. More women than men in the world. You too. Time will come.
> *Stephen*
> (Choking with fright, remorse, and horror) They said I killed you mother . . . Cancer did it, not I. Destiny.
> *The Mother*
> (A green rill of bile trickling from the side of her mouth) You sang that song to me. Love's bitter mystery.

It is here that we also learn about the more sinister side of the family unconscious. There is a sense of scarcity—not enough food, money, love, life, energy to go around to support everyone. The feeling of competitiveness is as old as Cain and Abel, and it is really at the sibling rivalry level in adult life that this is played out. The older legends are witness to scarcity. Abraham is ready to sacrifice Isaac. And Jesus is ready to die to save his family. There are few legends about having enough for everyone.

The importance of this stage of the family reunion is that upon the completion of mourning, the family consciously enters the unconscious state. Once this is achieved, it will be possible to modify the more primitive, rigid unconscious system with input from the higher aspects of our conscious selves.

3. Acknowledgment of the Paranoid Other

In Janet's family, the Wallachs prior to the meeting blamed their problems on the "damn doctor" who had not discovered Janet's tumor early enough. In Carla's family, it was the maid who was responsible for Carla's patterns of behavior. The maid, who had brought up Carla and her twin brother, was one day found hallucinating that worms were coming out of her nose as she watched the TV set. But the extended family finally acknowledged their own blame, for they all knew of this behavior, and had even used the maid after discovering her psychosis. (This was the same maid that one family had brought to dinner and was rejected by the other family.) As this part of the discussion went on, six members of Carla's family developed chest pains and Carla began to lose hers.

In my own family, there was considerable reality in the family paranoia about the "goyim," for the family had experienced a pogrom in every generation beginning from 1870, and half the family died in the Holocaust. Yet until this point, little had been said about the cohesiveness of the family during these trying times. My aunt Bella said that in Auschwitz and in the ghettos, families disintegrated because fathers took the food rations from their own children. The only unit you could count on was mother and child. Not even sister and sister.

4. Resolution

In the family reunion, you know you are progressing toward resolution when "triangulation" of communication stops. When communication is detriangled, as Bowen says, you make the situation less intense emotionally, and more stable. It is safer to talk about other people or things or concepts than each other.

With the beginning of dyadic communication, the resolution of problems is heralded by a separation of the generations. In Carla's family, she and her twin brother, her mother, and her grandmother were deeply involved in a single emotional system. One would start a sentence, the second would continue it, and the third would finish it. All four would mouth the script simultaneously, while one spoke for all. There was a tremendous amount of pain expressed as the separation began to occur. The mother was under the greatest pressure, as she also had to separate from her analyst at the meeting, as well as deal with the fact that Carla and her twin brother were about to leave home for college, leaving the parents alone for the first time since the children came.

In Janet's family, I am afraid that mother and daughter have not yet separated, although Kay, the younger daughter, seems to be better now. But it is as if the two—Janet and her mother—are living from the same energy. I worry about this, because even though there have been two subsequent meetings of the entire extended family, we have not cleared the system of its anger—this was glossed over by the immediate family. I worry also because plans for the wedding of Janet and her fiancé have recurred, and evidence of pressure in the family system is present: the father has returned to heavy drinking.

Before the point of separation of generations, the family may make a last-ditch effort to resist change. Here I have experienced tremendous anger directed at the therapist. As separation begins, I have also seen emotions get out of control. To an outsider, things would look completely crazy. A father rolls his daughter in the snow outside the meeting room. People walk around speaking to themselves. Someone may be screaming. It is important for the therapist to allow this disorganized behavior to continue, for it is likely to be short-lived. It is at this point that the family enters its most creative phase. The disorganized behavior is evidence of the separation that is occurring, the loss of old roles and identities, and the assuming of new roles as many members of the family come in contact more deeply with themselves.

It was at this point in the family reunion that Carla and her twin brother went into a birth agony. I went along with this simulated birth; Carla and her brother were experiencing a profound regression. Suddenly the family remembered what until that time had been blocked: that Carla's sternum had been crushed in the birth process and had to be supported by sutures for a few days afterward while she was in an incubator. I believed that her current separation pain, triggered by leaving home for college, was held in, resulting in the kind of chest pain she experienced at birth. This time her mother was able to relieve the pain, rubbing some soothing lotion lovingly on her daughter's chest.

In my own family reunion, although I remained silent for a while I could hear my own thoughts expressed by other members of the family in exactly the way I would have expressed them. It was a timeless state; I remember looking at my watch and noticing that only a few minutes had passed while it seemed we had been together for hours. The interaction process went deeper and deeper, and as the separation occurred things became simpler and problems became easier to manage.

Interestingly enough, in the family reunion, there is little sleep and little need for it. The physical movements of the family members become synchronized—it is as if the family has become a single organism, like an ameba. One person can speak for all, for the family members have introjected each other.

In the usual forms of family contact, or even in conventional family therapy, there is sufficient time between meetings to get the other family members out of your system. But in this kind of marathon meeting, family members are forced to take each other in, and they must digest and assimilate what they have incorporated. In this timeless state, where the family seems to have stepped out of life, the members watch their own behavior like actors in a play. In Carla's family, her aunt said, "My God, we are repeating a family script over and over."

5. The Creative Self

When the family is sharing this sense of oneness followed by the separation of generations, it is then that individual family members can become more fully in touch with themselves. Their language becomes eloquent, and it is a moving experience to see family members reveal themselves so honestly to one another. The facade people usually present, along with the defenses, is gone, and family members present themselves to others as they really are.

Family members begin to take risks and share fantasies they had never dared to reveal before. A physician says he wants to give up his busy practice to try his hand at filmmaking—not to be a great filmmaker, but just to try full-time something he loves doing. A housewife wants to become a therapist. A cancer victim wants to marry and have a child. At this level, everything seems possible. For the climate now is warm and loving, and there seems to be support from the rest of the family to try something new. Even overcoming cancer does not seem to be insurmountable. The family discovers solutions where no solutions appeared possible before.

About this time in the families I have dealt with, the life stories begin. For the family is acutely aware of the brevity of a lifetime, and the younger generations want to know in great detail about the lives of the older generations. In my family, the children learned about the pogrom in 1903, and about how it was possible to survive without clothes, money, or knowing the native language during World War II. These stories are the family mythology, which everyone strains to assimilate. I think the great success of *Roots* is no accident, for many people to reconnect in some way with the warmth that lies buried in all family systems.

6. The Aftermath

Like all peak experiences, the family reunion is followed by the inevitable let-down. I certainly found it a high point of my life. For months afterward, I lost the paranoid framework that my family had passed down to me about the way the world was, and I had a wonderful time finding my own way.

But soon after these meetings triangulation begins again, and some of the old issues which looked as if they had been resolved resurface. At this point I realized that the family reunion was only the beginning of a process. But the family had learned enough from the experience to know that even without a therapist we could again work toward a level of openness sufficient enough to deal better with the old problems and the new ones that inevitably appear. Since the original family reunion, my extended family has had another, briefer meeting without a therapist. At this meeting, 20 more members of the extended family participated than had been at the earlier meeting. We are planning yet another meeting soon. These meetings tend to occur around the natural events that bring families together—Thanksgivings, weddings, and so on.

Six months after the Alberts' family reunion Carla is at school, doing well, having worked through many of the issues raised at the meeting with her own therapist. Her mother is in the final phase of therapy and is now struggling with career goals. Six years after our first contact with the Wallach family, Janet is fully ambulatory, at school, and again engaged to be married. There have been two day-long meetings with 60 members of the extended family. But I am concerned about what will happen as Janet's wedding approaches again.

The family reunion is the beginning of an exploration into a very old form of healing, used by all groups in touch with their tribal roots, but nonetheless new to our society and our time. This is the first time in our history that the extended family has been so disrupted and there exists, I am convinced, the widespread phenomenon of individuals needing to reconnect with their extended families in some way—if not in the rigid way of the past.

In addition to the focus on families with a presenting emotional problem, I am carrying out family reunions on families with a high incidence of malignancy, heart disease, diabetes, and other kinds of illnesses of a genetic or familial origin. Most interesting in terms of prevention, is to meet with families before they enter the usual transitions: adolescence for the youngest generation, mid-life crisis for the parent generation, retirement for the grandparents, and dying for the grandparents, to use these predictable life crises for the promotion of the positive aspects of health.

FOOTNOTES

1. The name "Lamed Vovnik" was suggested to me by Dr. Charles Goodrich.

REFERENCES

Katz, R. Education for transcendence: !Kia-healing with the Kalahari !Kung, in Lee, R. and DeVore, I., eds. *Man the hunter.* Chicago, Ill.: Aldine Atherton, 1968.

Lee, R. *The !Kung San!: Men, women and work in a foraging society.* Cambridge, Great Britain: Cambridge University Press, 1979.

LeShan, L. Physicists and mystics: Similarities in world view. *Journal of Transpersonal Psychiatry,* 1969a, *1*(2).

LeShan, L. *Toward a general theory of the paranormal.* New York: Parapsychology Foundation, 1969b.

Rueveni, U. *Networking families in crisis.* New York: Human Sciences Press, 1979.

Speck, R. and Attneave, C. *Family networks.* New York: Pantheon Press, 1973.

Speck, R. and Rueveni, U. *Treating the family in times of crisis.* Current psychiatric therapies, 1977, *17*, 135–142.

Part III

INTERVENTIONS WITH FAMILIES
AND EXTENDED FAMILY SYSTEMS

Chapter 7

HEALING INTERVENTIONS WITH FAMILIES IN CRISIS

Uri Rueveni, Ph.D.

Family therapy and network therapy are viewed by Uri Rueveni as an intervention process. In this chapter the author describes his work with both members of the nuclear family and with the extended system in an effort to heal emotional crisis. Through the use of case material he describes strategies used with families focusing on the "death scene" as one effective strategy for healing.

Network intervention is viewed by the author as an extension of family therapy. Team development, home visits, the main network sessions, and follow-up support groups are described as well as the six network phases critical for the unfolding network process. The reader becomes familiar with the network approach and the identifiable roles of the intervention team by the use of vignettes from actual network intervention cases.

One definition of healing is to overcome, to restore to original integrity, to return to a sound state. Family members in an emotional crisis experience the strife, the hurt, the isolation, and lack of strength to cope with their dysfunctional relationships and life pressures. Such family members need indeed to be able to increase their ability to cope, to overcome, to restore their strength, to change—to heal.

Although there are a variety of forms in which families in our own culture have developed to heal themselves, this chapter addresses itself only to two specific interventions of healing families in emotional crisis. These are: *(1)* the development of some intervention strategies which can help family members cope better with life, and *(2)* the mobilizing of the extended family and social network for additional support of crisis resolution.

FAMILY THERAPY AS AN INTERVENTION STRATEGY

Family therapy can be viewed as an intervention process. It can become a more effective intervention process when members of the ailing family allow the therapist to intervene in an attempt to help them regain increased confidence, competence, and strength in utilizing their resources to overcome the crisis, to change and heal.

In the last two decades the field of family therapy has been growing and an increased number of both theoretical frameworks and clinical approaches have been formulated. The reader should familiarize himself with the following important contributions: Ackerman, 1966; Alger, 1976; Auerswald, 1972; Bandler, Grinder, and Satir, 1976; Bell, 1975; Bloch and LePerriere, 1973; Boszormenyi-Nagy and Spark, 1973; Bowen, 1966, 1978; Duhl, Kantor, and Duhl, 1973; Ferber, 1972; Framo, 1965, 1975; Haley, 1976; Jackson, 1965; Minuchin, 1978; Napier and Whitaker, 1972, 1978; Satir, 1967; Speck, 1964, 1967; Whitaker, 1978; Zuk, 1971.

To most families an emotional crisis is experienced as a threat and some family members have been to individual therapy, or sought help from numerous other sources within their family and community systems prior to contacting a family therapist. When the family therapist becomes involved with family work he/she is facing numerous issues already in operation within the family which may have to be addressed and worked through. Such issues as ineffective and often destructive communication patterns, eroding trust levels among family members, hidden agendas, family secrets, excessive enmeshments between parents and children, and a host of other related issues all can contribute to the maintenance of the dysfunctional family patterns, some of which will need to be dealt with if family healing is to take place.

Although there are available today a variety of approaches which attempt to help the family therapist deal with some of these issues, I am most comfortable in the framework which allows me to function as a strategist for change (Rueveni, 1979). This concept implies that the family therapist becomes involved with a family system in a human and caring way, attempting to help family members change their dysfunctional pattern of relationships by utilizing a wide variety of techniques and approaches which will allow for change in the relationships among the members.

Developing Intervention Strategies

Family therapy sessions can present the therapists with ample opportunities for effective interventions. Effective intervention strategies, in my opinion, are those which are based on the therapist's observations of the interaction among family members which foster and maintain continued problems and dysfunctions.

My own intervention strategies result primarily from impressions which I form about the relationship among the family members. I view myself as a consultant to the family, but I am not always objective, nor do I pretend to be. I take sides often, making sure that each family member has an opportunity to be supported by me at one time or another. To me, side-taking is only one of many of the intervention strategies I am willing to use for achieving change, relief of family discomfort, and greater family harmony. My choices of an intervention strategy are basically eclectic, and vary from being a go-between and side-taker (Zuk, 1975), to the use of family sculpting (Papp, 1976), and psychodramatic approaches to the mobilization of an entire family network to abate a family crisis and find alternatives for family coping (Rueveni, 1979).

As a strategist for change, the family therapist is actively involved in engaging family members to examine their relationships and seek alternative ways of coping with one another. To help the family members achieve these changes requires the therapist to activate his/her experiences, timing his/her responses, and stimulating activities or the lack of them, in appropriate timing sequences.

Whether I see the family in my office or in their own home, I can function best when I am me, allowing myself to be transparent and self-disclosing, when appropriate. I find it most useful to relate to family members in the first person, and to communicate my feelings and thoughts directly. In any initial session, I attempt to lay out the ground rules for our future meetings, which are, that I will work with the family as long as I feel I can be useful in helping them change. I usually meet the family for an hour-and-a-half session on a weekly basis, for a period of ten to fifteen sessions. I encourage the married children to bring in their spouses. When some family members absent themselves regularly from the session, I often suggest conducting the therapy in their own home or apartment.

My strategy with absent members is to call them first, letting them know that I would like them to continue coming. If resistance continues, I encourage the remaining members to continually "leak" information which directly concerns the absent members and which usually triggers a telephone call by them to me, at which point I encourage their participation, if for nothing else, at least to defend the "good name" they think they deserve. As for the home meetings, I try to keep those to a minimum, and prefer them only when the larger network extended system is mobilized.

I find that family members' perception of me varies from being a mentor, consultant, and advisor, to a friend, a parent, a family member, and a caring person. Becoming engaged in the process of helping the family change, I allow myself to be touched emotionally so that I find myself soft-spoken, tender, and loving with one family member, angry at times with another, still hurt by another, crying when I need to, laughing with the family when it is time to laugh, and sharing a story when it seems appropriate to do so.

I consider my authenticity an important part of the intervention process. As Framo (1975) has suggested: The willingness to reveal oneself is often the catalyst for establishing important human contact with a patient or a family.

With families where I can develop trust rapidly, I can speed up my intervention. On the other hand, where trust and credibility are slower to develop, I attempt to assess the family readiness for an intervention which I may want to suggest. I stress that the sense of timing of an intervention strategy is quite important, and therapists can gain it mostly by experiences and willingness to learn what strategy produces productive changes among family members.

The "Death Scene"—A Strategic Technique for Change

In the following similar case, I attempt to demonstrate one strategic technique I have used with some families to speed up the process of greater family involvement, and hopefully, initiating the possibilities of problem solving, reduction in crisis, and change in the system. I do not see it as a "cure-all" but only as one strategy at my disposal, to be used when appropriate.

This technique explores the issue of loss and death in the family system. I find that with many dysfunctional family systems it is useful to introduce this issue by encouraging one family member to close his/her eyes, lie down on a chair or the floor, and pretend he/she is dead, while other family members "eulogize" the "dead" family member. I have used this experience in both family therapy context and within the larger family network experience and found it to be helpful, giving the family a unique opportunity for feeling closer to each other and sharing feelings which are positive and productive for further healing.

Case 1. A 27-year-old woman was referred for severe depression and ongoing threats to take her own life. In family therapy, attended by her husband, both of her parents, her married brother, and his spouse, a sad story unfolded. How the young woman could not accept the shape of her buttocks and constantly sought surgery to change their shape. In family therapy, the focus of the sessions was rarely on the suicide attempt or the surgery, but instead focused on the relationship between father and daughter. Father, acting and looking like Archie Bunker, was blamed by his daughter for abusing her mentally while she was growing up. Father seemed to be making most of the decisions at home and I knew I had to gain his confidence and trust first. Our initial encounter occurred in the beginning of the first session. He came in wanting to know what I thought about Archie Bunker. My reply was that I had gotten to know him as a human being, and I shared with father my feelings about the scene from the television series where Archie and "Meathead," his son-in-law, were stuck in the basement all night and the tender feelings Archie was able to share with "Meathead" about his own childhood and his relationship with his own father. The patient's father's eyes lit up and he smiled, reaching the chair, and sitting comfortably. I knew from that moment on, I could communicate with him, respecting each other's right to be different. As I proceeded with this family, working on the relationships, my main goal was to have father and daughter achieve a degree of closeness they had never had before.

During the third session, the young woman verbally abused her father, wishing he were dead for all the agony he had given her when she was a growing girl. I felt it to be an appropriate time for intervention on my part. I decided to ask her father to consider himself dead, close his eyes, and lie down on the couch. He agreed, and his daughter proceeded to eulogize him, at my request, as the rest of the family sat sobbing. The daughter knelt at her father's feet and began to apologize, and sobbingly shared, for the first time, her feelings of love for him and wishing to be closer to him.

This experience provided the beginning of the healing I was hoping for: following this session, the suicide threats stopped, replaced with a more open sharing by all family members, about the kind of activities they could begin to become engaged with in the near future, in an attempt to improve their relationships.

Case 2. As we all have experienced, success in working with the entire family is not always possible. I have had my share of frustrations in expecting the entire family to continually come to therapy or in stopping such "favorite" family activities as scapegoating, collusions, triangulations, and enmeshments.

The following case began with the entire family system coming for therapy and upon termination, only the female family members remained.

A family of eight was referred to me in an attempt to help their 14-year-old daughter, Susan, overcome her school phobia and return to her classroom. The initial session revealed quite a dysfunctional family system, consisting of an alcoholic father, an overweight and physically ill (heart problems) mother, their 13-year-old, blind son, reported to be acting out in school, plus a 17-year-old, pregnant daughter in her last year of high school. There were also two married children, one, a 30-year-old son who came to the session with his wife. She reported that her husband was unemployed, drank heavily, and was physically abusing her. The other was a 23-year-old daughter who came by herself since her husband was having recurrent problems with epileptic seizures.

Susan, the school-phobic daughter, was perceived by all family members as having "the problem," and their attendance in family therapy was to help her go back to school. In addition, mother felt that Susan utters "strange" sounds during the night, and the suggestions that came from other family members were, that perhaps Susan had a "multiple personality" problem.

I encouraged all family members to consider the possibility that they were all in therapy to help each other relate better and this might help Susan return to school. Although the first session seemed to be involving everyone, the male members of the family refused to return and become involved further with family therapy, claiming they were all busy at work. I chose to continue working with the female members while urging the men to return as soon as possible. The remaining sessions were attended by mother and her daughters. All five felt abandoned by men and felt they needed strength in order to live their daily lives. At one point in the session, mother expressed her wish to die, stating that in the past she thought of walking by the railroad tracks, wishing the train would pass and kill her instantly. Her daughters disclosed that when their mother was hospitalized recently, they were quite distressed, fearing she might die and wishing to die with her. My strategy at this point was to give the opportunity to the daughters to express their feelings for their own mother. I asked mother to pretend she was dead, and the ensuing event was one of the most moving experiences I have witnessed. All the daughters, crying and sharing with their mother their love and affection over the years for her stating that they were never able to let her know how they really felt about her.

During the following session, Susan was making plans to return to school with the help of her sisters and the school counselor offered an opportunity to begin completing the missing work at her office, gradually easing Susan back into the classroom. Susan's fears of having her mother die by suicide or by being physically abused by her own father, began to lose strength and were replaced by openness and support, primarily from her own mother, who felt that she now had a reason to exist and to return the love expressed toward her by her daughters. Again, in this case, not all the problems were solved in the family. However, the main goal of having Susan return to school was achieved. My frequent follow-ups with the family indicated continued progress in the relationships between family members, including the male members of the family.

Case 3. Mrs. K. came to see me by herself, claiming she was depressed, not loved or understood by her husband and her two younger children, a boy eleven and a girl thirteen. I wanted to see the entire family but Mrs. K. balked at first, claiming her husband would not come under any circumstances. My first strategy was to ask her to give him my card and ask him to make the appointment. He did and when they came together, the husband said that this was his first and last visit unless his wife would resume sex with him immediately. I replied that I did not really care if he did not continue coming because it would give me an opportunity to fall in love with her. Needless to say, he was quite furious and said he would not return. However, as expected, at the next appointment the entire family came and we began the process of becoming involved with the business at hand.

The most important issue in this family relationship was father's absence and the resentment his wife and children had concerning his taking more time to be with them. These issues did not surface until a later session. At one point, the wife stated that her husband was dead for all practical purposes. I decided to ask her husband to pretend he was dead. When he did so, it provided a new opportunity to communicate at a different level for all family members, and rekindled memories by the husband about his own life at home and his own feelings of being abandoned by his parents, acknowledging the similarities in this pattern. I felt that this experience provided again the turning point in this family's struggle to increase communication and begin to alleviate some of the pain in their strained relationships.

MOBILIZING THE FAMILY'S SOCIAL SUPPORT NETWORK

The literature on family and social networks has been steadily growing and professionals from the disciplines of anthropology, sociology, psychology, psychiatry, and related fields have contributed to an increased understanding of the field (Attneave, 1969; Barnes, 1972; Bott, 1971; Cohen and Sokolovsky, 1978; Collins and Pancoast, 1976; Curtis, 1973; Erickson, 1975; Garrison, 1974, 1976; Gatti, 1976; Hammer, 1963; Hansell, 1967; Pattison, 1973, 1975; Rueveni, 1975, 1976, 1977, 1979; Rueveni and Speck, 1969; Sarason, 1977; Speck, 1967; Speck and Rueveni, 1969; Speck and Attneave, 1973; Speck and Speck, 1979; Todd, 1979; Tolsdorf, 1976.

An excellent summary of all network approaches practiced today was written by Trimble (1980). The reader is advised to familiarize himself with these important contributions to the field of networks.

The view taken here is that most families need to be able to maintain an ongoing relationship with their extended family and social network. The importance of connecting with extended kin network as well as with one's own social/community system cannot be overemphasized. The fact that many families are unable or unwilling to continue their relationships and maintain an active connection with their extended family system serves as a sad commentary on our current lifestyle, culture, and value system.

Family therapists need to be able to increasingly involve the extended family system in their therapeutic efforts. As Attneave (1980) suggests, social networks are a logical extension of family therapy. Dysfunctional families in crisis need to be able to reactivate many sources of strengths and to infuse their system with new energies and fresh ideas. The energy available within one's own family and social system, if mobilized, can be channeled toward family healing and crisis resolution.

The Network Stages and Phases

There are basically four main stages to any attempt of full-scale mobilization of one's own family network. The first stage is team development, the second is the home visit, the third is the main sessions with all the family and social network in attendance, and the fourth stage is the support group follow-up. Each of these stages is important to the successful mobilization of the entire network.

Team Development.   Any efforts at working with 40 or more extended family members are best achieved by the selection of a team of family interventionists. The team should be as small as two or as large as four or five members. A good team should consist of a leader who is seasoned in working with families, and has experience in group dynamics. Other team members should have experience in working with families or groups and be able to feel comfortable with large group experiences. Skills in psychodrama and group dynamics are quite helpful. The team should be able to work with and relate to each other well.

Since the network approach often requires team members to work at odd hours, spending time in planning pre- and postfamily session strategies, they must be willing to invest a great deal of energy with family members who need the "extra push" to change. The team leadership could rotate; however, during the network sessions it is best if one leader conducts the sessions with assistance and consultation from teammates.

The Home Visit.   Members of the intervention team need to become familiar with the family's concerns and the appropriateness of conducting the full-scale network assembly. When one works with the family for a while and gets to know their concerns, the need for a home visit may not be as critical as when the family is a new referral. The best way to assess the appropriateness of mobilizing the network assembly with a new referral is to meet with members of the family at their home. The meeting usually produces a host of data needed for a decision to mobilize the network.

During such a meeting, team members are interested in the family's previous efforts at seeking help for solving their problems. They need to have a "feel" for the family's dysfunction. They need to become familiar with each of the family member's concerns and their readiness to participate in activating the network. The team members do not necessarily seek a consensus of opinion. In fact, it is a rare occasion when all family members can agree about inviting their entire network of family and friends for such a meeting. However, the team strategy during this stage is to "seek out" allies within the family who would be willing to risk, to become involved, to reach out to their extended system in their time of crisis.

The team members need to encourage the "family activists" who often need just this opportunity to be given to them to speak out and lead others in their family to take this additional step so important for their healing.

The decision to mobilize the network then rests on a host of issues. The most important criterion is the family's degree of desperation. We often find that the more desperate the crisis, the more agreeable members of the family are to mobilize their network. Other important criteria are the availability of a sufficient number of family and friends. There are some occasions when one finds it very difficult to mobilize more than ten people. However, experience indicates that most families, if motivated to do so, can easily call upon at least 40 or more of their family and friends to participate.

Another factor in mobilizing the network is the ease with which members of the family will allow themselves to trust each other, the team, and others in their system to become involved in the networking process. This process requires a high degree of family involvement, a willingness to open up one's own "can of worms," and to discuss family secrets and relationships which could be of some embarrassment to one's own family and friends.

The Main Network Meeting, Network Phases, and Team Strategies.   A successful mobilization of the family network process usually unfolds into six distinct phases. The first phase is *retribalization*, an initial period where network members begin to reconnect with each other. During this phase, the team members encourage the participants to mill around and meet as many people as possible. Some group activities can also be suggested such as singing a song, swaying, and humming and similar activities which will allow for the network participants to mobilize energies involving themselves as a more cohesive group.

The next phase is that of *polarization*. During this phase, participants exchange differing points of view regarding the problems in the family. This polarization is important since it involves others in the network with the different issues which need to be addressed. The team leader needs to allow this expression of different points of view and attempts to inhibit it will make progress difficult.

Mobilization is the next phase. During this period some people in the network begin to mobilize themselves, take leadership positions, and offer ideas which may lead to the reduction of the crisis. The team continues to encourage further exploration of all aspects of the family's concerns.

The phase of *depression* usually follows. During this phase many people begin to express frustration at their inability to help. Others feel that the problems are too difficult and they cannot be of help. The task of the intervention team is to acknowledge the difficulties but to insist on the collective ability of the network to solve the crisis. The team leader can usually activate the network into action by choreographing some strategic move, usually a psychodramatic experience, which will allow family members and others in the network to become further involved with the difficult issues at hand.

The final two phases are *breakthrough* and *exhaustion elation*. During these two phases some solutions and alternatives seem to begin to be formulated. The team strategy is to encourage the development and formation of support groups and the feeling on the part of many in the network is that of exhaustion, but also of elation, a feeling of some accomplishment and the ability that positive changes in the family may be forthcoming as a result of their efforts.

The Support Groups.   The last stage of the network is the formation of the support groups around each of the family members. The team strategy is to mobilize members of the network to form small support groups of at least five to 15 people who will meet with any of the family members who feel they can use the network support. The support group members need to activate their resources and organize themselves in a manner which will allow for ongoing and continuous weekly meetings with members of the family for at least a number of weeks until the immediate crisis can be reduced and the alternative solutions which were formulated in the initial main session can be carried out.

The Roles of the Network Therapist.   There are specific and identifiable roles which the network therapist and members of the team undertake during each network intervention session. These roles are: convenor, mobilizer, choreographer, and resource consultant.

The Therapist as a Convenor.   The therapist and the team function as network convenors primarily during the home visit and the retribalization phase.

During a home visit to a black family struggling with a son who had been previously hospitalized for psychiatric episodes and who exhibited an enmeshed relationship to his mother, members of the team helped the family to chart a family tree and prepare a list of invited guests.

With another family, a mother struggling to cope with two emotionally disturbed daughters, the team helped to convene 40 network participants who came for a workshop and became involved in a live demonstration of the process by participating as active members.

A young woman hospitalized in an adolescent unit of a psychiatric hospital needed to attend the home meeting with her family; the team arranged with the unit's director to allow for her participation, and the convening of the first family network was coordinated by the team to coincide with the day of the young woman's release from the hospital.

A network meeting was about to begin in another family home in an attempt to help both parents cope with their 20-year-old daughter who had barricaded herself in the vestibule, refusing to leave it or to eat or sleep. Since only a small number of people showed up for the first network meeting, the team members, with the family's permission, went outside the house and recruited and convened additional neighbors and members of the nearby church, including the minister who was familiar with the family's ongoing concerns.

It should be emphasized that the family members take the initiative and responsibility of calling on their support system for help. However, the therapist and the team clearly function as convenors particularly as the full-scale network convenes.

The role of the network therapist during the retribalization phase is to allow network members to increase their energy "level" and their readiness for further involvement with the family. The network team functions as family convenors by leading the entire assembly in a sequence of activities such as singing a favorite family melody in unison, or milling around, meeting people, holding hands in a circle, swaying, to name just a few. These activities allow for a greater group readiness and prepare the network for its difficult task of becoming involved with the family's problems.

During one network meeting, assembled to stop a young woman's suicidal attempts and provide alternative ways of coping by all family members, the entire network convened and sang the melody Sunrise Sunset from "Fiddler on the Roof." Both parents began to sob and the mother was held by her husband as the rest of the network members were getting ready to deal with the unfolding family problem.

In another network during a Friday night meeting with a Jewish family designed to help family members deal with their son's ongoing depressions, the role of convening the network became easier when one cousin, a rabbinical student, agreed to lead the participants in the traditional Jewish ceremony of lighting the candles and offering the blessing welcoming the Sabbath.

Zuk (1975) suggests that the therapist function as a celebrant at times. The healing ceremony of the !Kung/Zhan/Twasi as described by Katz (1976) involved a whole community dance activity which is aimed at the release of energy and healing. The retribalization phase then offers the network team a chance to function in the role of convenors of the family network assembly, allowing for the proper unfolding of the remaining network phases.

The Network Therapist as a Mobilizer. The mobilization of the network for action can be achieved by the ongoing involvements of the network members in the ongoing struggles of the family. Both family and network members need to be able to actively participate in sharing and disclosing thoughts and feelings, exchanging different points of view, and continuously and actively engaging in the networking process.

The mobilization phase of each network is usually characterized by the formation of the network activists. These are the members within the family and the extended family network who are willing to reactivate additional energies and efforts, demonstrating leadership qualities in helping solve the family crisis.

During the mobilization phase as well as during the next phase of depression, where feelings of frustration are increasing, the network therapist and team are engaged in a role best described as a mobilizer. They need to encourage participants to try harder, and they need to help keep the dialogue and exchange of feelings and thoughts remaining at an active level. In short, the need is to keep the network mobilized. A few vignettes of this role follow:

During a network assembled to help a young man find alternatives to his use of drugs, his uncle indicated that there are problems galore in the family. His wife and other family members ignored his comments. However, the team leader insisted that he clarify his statement, which revealed that an important and active family member (the young man's aunt) was not invited to attend since she uses drugs and was believed to be a bad influence on the family. The insistence of the team on dealing with this issue helped the network become mobilized around the issues of drug use and abuse, scapegoating, and on the relationships that existed between the young man and his parents.

In another network assembled to provide support for crisis resolution for a divorced woman, her five children and her 14-year-old psychotic daughter, the latter refused to attend the meeting, hid in the garage, and tied herself to the door with a rope. During the network meeting, one team member found a note in the girl's bedroom demanding to be considered as a sane person, requesting a change in her school, and privileges which if granted would stop her "bizarre" behavior. The efforts of the team were directed toward mobilizing the network to consider the letter. Some network activists were able to encourage the young girl to leave the garage and stay in the basement where communication developed between herself and her family and also with her activist support group.

The Network Therapist as a Choreographer. The therapist and his team need to be able to operate at two simultaneous levels during each network session: the nuclear family and the network system levels. To ensure continuous interaction between members of these two systems, and to facilitate the transition from one network phase to the other, the network team often functions as choreographers. Papp (1976) described this role as a method of actively intervening in the nuclear and extended family by realigning family relationships through physical and movement positioning.

During each network meeting the therapist and team need to undertake this role by developing active and dramatic approaches which will activate the network process. The role of the therapist as a choreographer often involves a variety of techniques and strategies including psychodramatic approaches, family sculpting and encounter techniques which can provide family members with an opportunity to begin and explore more supportive and trusting levels of their relationships.

A network meeting was assembled to help members of a family develop new strengths in dealing with an ongoing crisis: the death of their father. The mother, a woman in her fifties who had lost her husband, had increasing difficulty in relating to her 15-year-old daughter who had begun acting out intensely following her father's death. She began using drugs, attempted to set fire to the family home, and attempted to overdose frequently. Although this child was under psychiatric care on an outpatient basis, her behavior seemed to be rapidly deteriorating. Her two older brothers and one sister were married and living away from home. However, they were working in the same business and frequently rotated in having their younger sister visit them in their homes but finding the experience difficult to cope with. The relationships between the mother and all of her children remained stressful at best. During the network meeting the team strategy included an experience which would allow the young girl, as well as her family, to express their feelings of loss and mourning toward their recently deceased father. A choreographed move was designed whereby members of the nuclear family stood in a circle sending verbal "postcards" to their dead father, expressing their feelings toward him when he was alive, how much they missed him, and what commitment they could make to ensure that their lives without him could continue and get the family free from pain and strife. This experience provided an excellent opportunity for further network mobilization and involvement by the family and their support network.

Another choreographic move with the same family members occurred during the second meeting. Each of the family members sat by their mother and made individual pledges to improve their relationships by discussing ways of coping with the situation and exchanging feelings. At the conclusion of this experience, the mother remained in the middle of the circle, hugged by her inner family circle including her 15-year-old daughter and by the outer circle of all the network members, each taking their time to share and contribute to the events taking place.

In another network meeting to stop a suicidal attempt by a 25-year-old divorced woman whose relationship with her mother was very stressful, the therapist and team choreographed a psychodramatic event where the daughter was asked to step up on a chair, looking down toward her mother who was sitting. The daughter who previously felt helpless and controlled by her mother, was encouraged to communicate her feelings toward her mother. This initial confrontation provided the daughter with a new opportunity to express her feelings openly with the support of her sister and to begin the process of healing.

During a network meeting to help a mother begin the process of minimizing her enmeshment with her psychotic son, a mock funeral ceremony was conducted, the son was considered to be "dead," was covered up, and the mother proceeded to eulogize him. This choreographed experience provided a new opportunity for both mother and her family network to express their feelings toward the son and begin a healing process whereby the network support system could provide new alternative arrangements for a temporary separation between mother and son.

The Network Therapist as a Resource Consultant. The role of a resource consultant is undertaken by the network team primarily during the formation of the support groups. At this stage, team members usually provide initial leadership to the support group formation and composition. This role is also continued to be maintained as the network meetings are completed and is followed by the ongoing follow-up of the support group meetings with members of the family.

Toward the end of the sessions with one family, the network team remained active in helping to form a support group for the young daughter and for her mother. They provided consultations and offered ideas of additional resources to be explored by members of the support group. The daughter considered the team's suggestion to make arrangements for going back to school, for a part-time job, and for providing ongoing social contact during the week. The mother's support group helped her in forming new social contacts, and reopened new and old friendships resulting from the two network sessions.

In the network which met to help the enmeshed mother and her psychotic son, the therapist and the team were instrumental as resource consultants to the support groups. Following the second network meeting, the son was helped by his support group to take an apartment at the YMCA. He attempted to return home the following evening, only to find the locks changed. Mother's support group had provided her with the strength not to allow her son to return that evening. The son's support group was instrumental in encouraging him to visit his mother only on a weekly basis, to find a new job, and to stop his self-destructive behavior patterns. Members of the team kept in daily contact with each support group, offering suggestions and consultation on helping in the case, and helped with the disengagement process.

SUMMARY

I have attempted in this presentation to elucidate on my own approach with families in crisis. It is a goal-oriented, problem-solving approach, which allows the therapist to intervene in a dysfunctional family system by utilizing various intervention modalities to include mobilization of the entire family and social system. To be sure, there are many occasions where the therapist need not or could not activate the family system to become involved in the methods described in this chapter. Working with the family in crisis is no easy undertaking for any therapist. It can often be a demanding and frustrating experience if no change occurs in the system, and when the therapist feels helpless in helping the family members change.

The process of engaging the dysfunctional family in working through their often unexpressed and unresolved issues becomes a much more rewarding experience for both therapist and family members when trust develops between all concerned, when goals can be defined and redefined, and when the therapist and his team can function with both the family and its network in a more harmonious integrated way, helping the family members find alternative options of coping, changing, and healing.

REFERENCES

Ackerman, N. W. *Treating the troubled family.* New York: Basic Books, 1966.
Algar, I. Audio-visual techniques in family therapy, in Bloch, D. A., ed. *Techniques of family psychotherapy: A primer.* New York: Grune and Stratton, 1973.
Attneave, C. L. Therapy in tribal settings and urban network intervention. *Family Process,* 1969, *8,* 192–210.
Attneave, C. L. Social networks and clinical practice: A logical extension of family therapy, in Freeman, D. S., ed. *Perspectives on family therapy.* Vancouver, B. C.: Butterworth & Co., 1980.
Auerswald, E. H. Families, change, and the ecological perspective. *Family Process,* 1971, *10,* 263–280.
Bandler, R., Grinder, J., and Satir, V. *Changing with families.* Palo Alto, Calif.: Science and Behavior Books, 1976.
Barnes, J. Clan and committees in a Norwegian island parish. *Human Relations,* 1954, *7.*
Bell, J. E. *Family therapy.* New York: Jason Aronson, 1975.
Bloch, D. A. and La Perriere, K. Techniques of family therapy: A conceptual frame, in Bloch, D. A., ed. *Techniques of family psychotherapy: A primer.* New York: Grune and Stratton, 1973.
Boszormenyi-Nagy, I. and Spark, G. M. *Invisible loyalties: Reciprocity in intergenerational family therapy.* New York: Harper & Row, 1973.
Bott, E. *Family and social network* (second ed). London: Tavistock Publications, 1971.
Bowen, M. *Family therapy in clinical practice.* New York: Jason Aronson, 1978.
Cohen, C. I. and Sokolovsky, J. Schizophrenia and social networks: Ex-patients in the inner city. *Schizophrenia Bulletin,* 1978, *4,* 546–560.
Collins, A. H. and Pancoast, D. L. *Natural helping networks: A strategy for prevention.* Washington: National Association of Social Workers Publications, 1976.
Curtis, W. R. Community human service networks, new roles for mental health workers. *Psychiatric Annals,* 1973, *3,* 23–42.

Curtis, W. R. The future use of social networks in mental health, in Pattison, E. M. (Chair), *Clinical group methods for larger social systems.* Symposium presented at the 33rd Annual Conference of the American Group Psychotherapy Association, Boston, February 1976.

Duhl, F. J., Kantor, D., and Duhl, B. S. Learning, space, and action in family therapy: A primer of sculpture, in Bloch, D. A., ed. *Techniques of family psychotherapy: A primer.* New York: Grune and Stratton, 1973.

Erickson, C. E. The concept of personal network in clinical practice. *Family Process,* 1975, *14,* 487–498.

Ferber, A. and Ranz, J. How to succeed in family therapy: Set reachable goals—give workable tasks, in Sager, C. J. and Kaplan, H. S., eds. *Progress in group and family therapy.* New York: Brunner/Mazel, 1972.

Framo, J. L. Rationale and techniques of intensive family therapy, in Boszormenyi-Nagy, I. and Framo, J. L., eds. *Intensive family therapy: Theoretical and practical aspects.* New York: Harper & Row, 1965.

Framo, J. L. Personal reflections of a family therapist. *Journal of Marriage and Family Counseling,* 1975, *1,* 15–28.

Garrison, J. E. Network techniques: Case studies in the screening-linking-planning conference method. *Family Process,* 1974, *13,* 337–353.

Garrison, J. E. Network methods for clinical problems, in Pattison, E. M. (Chair), *Clinical group methods for larger social systems.* Symposium presented at the 33rd Annual Conference of the American Group Psychotherapy Association, Boston, February 1976.

Gatti, F. and Colman, C. Community network therapy: An approach to aiding families with troubled children. *American Journal of Orthopsychiatry,* 1976, *40,* 608–617.

Haley, J. *Problem-solving therapy.* San Francisco: Jossey-Bass, 1976.

Hammer, M. Influence of small social networks on factors in mental hospital admissions. *Human Organization,* 1963, *22,* 243–251.

Hansell, N. Patient predicament and clinical service: A system. *Archives of General Psychiatry,* 1967, *17,* 204–210.

Jackson, D. D. The study of the family. *Family Process,* 1965, *4,* 1–20.

Katz, R. The painful ecstasy of healing. *Psychology Today,* 1976, *10,* 81–96.

Minuchin, S., Rosman, B. L., and Baker, L. *Psychosomatic families: Anorexia nervosa in context.* Cambridge, Mass.: Harvard University Press, 1978.

Napier, A. Y. and Whitaker, C. A. A conversation about co-therapy, in Ferber, A., Mendelsohn, M., and Napier, A. Y., eds. *The book of family therapy.* New York: Science House, 1972.

Napier, A. Y. and Whitaker, C. A. *The family crucible.* New York: Harper & Row, 1978.

Papp, P. Family choreography, in Guerin, P. G., Jr., ed. *Family therapy: Theory and practice.* New York: Gardiner Press, 1976.

Pattison, E. M. Social system psychotherapy. *American Journal of Psychotherapy,* 1973, *18,* 396–409.

Pattison, E. M., DeFrancisco, D., Wood, W., Frazier, H., and Crowder, J. A psychosocial kinship model for family therapy. *American Journal of Psychiatry*, 1975, *132*, 1246–1251.

Rueveni, U. Network intervention with a family crisis. *Family Process*, 1975, *14*, 193–204.

Rueveni, U. Family network intervention: Healing families in crisis. *Intellect*, 1976, May-June, pp. 580–582.

Rueveni, U. Family network intervention: Mobilizing support for families in crisis. *International Journal of Family Counseling*, 1977, *5*, 77–83.

Rueveni, U. *Networking families in crisis*. New York: Human Sciences Press, 1979.

Rueveni, U. and Speck, R. V. Using encounter group techniques in the treatment of the social network of the schizophrenic. *International Journal of Group Psychotherapy*, 1969, *19*, 495–500.

Rueveni, U. and Wiener, M. Network intervention of disturbed families: The key role of network activists. *Psychotherapy: Theory, Research and Practice*, December 1976, *13*, 173–176.

Sarason, S. B., Carroll, C. F., Maton, K. Cohen, S., and Lorentz, E. *Human services and resource networks*. San Francisco: Jossey-Bass, 1977.

Satir, V. *Conjoint family therapy: A guide to theory and technique*. Palo Alto, Calif.: Science and Behavior Books, 1967.

Speck, R. V. Family therapy in the home. *Journal of Marriage and Family Living*, 1964, *26*, 72–76.

Speck, R. V. Psychotherapy of the social network of a schizophrenic family. *Family Process*, 1967, *7*, 208–214.

Speck, R. V. and Attneave, C. L. *Family networks*. New York: Pantheon Books, 1973.

Speck, R. V. and Rueveni, U. Network therapy: A developing concept. *Family Process*, 1969, *8*, 182–191.

Speck, R. V. and Speck, J. L. On networks: Network therapy, network intervention and networking. *International Journal of Family Therapy*, Winter, 1979, pp. 333–337.

Todd, D. M. Social networks and psychology. *Connections*, Spring, 1979, *2(2)*, 87–88.

Tolsdorf, C. C. Social networks, support, and coping: An exploratory study. *Family Process*, 1976, *15*, 407–417.

Trimble, D. A guide to the network therapies. 1980, unpublished paper.

Whitaker, C. A. Cotherapy of chronic schizophrenia, in Berger, M. ed. *Beyond the double bind: Communication and family systems, theories and techniques with schizophrenics*. New York: Brunner/Mazel, 1978.

Zuk, G. H. *Family therapy: A triadic-based approach*. New York: Human Sciences Press, 1971.

Zuk, G. H. *Process and practice in family therapy*. Haverford, Pa.: Psychiatry and Behavioral Sciences Books, 1975.

Chapter 8

CRISIS INTERVENTION WITH MEXICAN-AMERICAN FAMILIES AND EXTENDED FAMILIES

Edmundo J. Ruiz, M.D.

The emphasis of this chapter is in defining and recognizing the total social matrix in a given cultural situation. Edmundo Ruiz demonstrates here that the constructs and context of the Mexican-American family have significantly different emphases in the function of the family and extended family's social structure. In crisis intervention, defined as goal-oriented rather than toward basic personality change, built-in systems of mutuality—reciprocity and obligation—must be utilized. This he portrays in three sensitive vignettes, each using variations of social network intervention and healing.

Human healing systems today are confronted with more crisis intervention than a few decades ago. The rapid changes and threatening events around the world at this time have added the pressure of giving attention to crisis, and have caused an upsurge in public, professional, and official governmental interest in crisis intervention programs and/or techniques.

"The family's emotional reactions to crisis, and the helper's own reactions when confronted with these problems, are the subject of this chapter. The therapist finds himself under pressure to help solve the family's problems, both conscious and unconscious, since they are presented in the heightened emotional setting of a major family crisis. He too, has his own reactions, both conscious and unconscious, to the family and the crisis; a family who not only expects to have the answers to its crisis, but also to have something done immediately." (Group for the Advancement of Psychiatry, 1963)

"Stress is normal, inevitable, a part of life. It is experienced in family relationships, school, work, traffic, shopping, financial, and in other problems. Everyone develops means of coping more or less effectively. Some means of coping are beneficial as, for example, when the response is an effort to improve performance. But there are destructive responses such as excessive alcohol use, drugs, violence, reckless behavior, depression, and other forms of mental illness" HEW; 1969.

It has been proved that stress is also the precipitating factor of somatic disorders, or proneness to illness, or changes in body functions; but if stress, or an individual's reaction to it, is excessive, physiological changes can be so dramatic as to have serious physical and emotional consequences. Considering all this, the goal should be to prevent or reduce destructive stress, and to help develop the individual's skills in coping with it.

"What is a crisis? It is an emotionally significant event, or radical change of status in a person's life which is disruptive of his usual mode of adaptation" (Amada, 1977). In crisis, intervention is essentially time-limited, or crisis-oriented, which signifies fewer sessions—fewer than nine—and requires a fast, practical, and concrete response to the situation and an immediate psychological relief, not a basic personality transformation. It is ordinarily sensible and therapeutic to regard any reason a psychiatric client employs for seeking psychotherapy, as a legitimate expression of a personal crisis which requires prompt psychotherapeutic help.

> Crisis intervention is a well conceptualized process of short term psychotherapy, based on the assumption that persons are amenable to therapeutic intervention and adaptive change at the perceived crisis. Treatment is goal-oriented—goals focused on the rapid mobilization of the individual's emotional resources to resolve the immediate psychological crisis, the restoration of a precrisis level of functioning, and the development of more adaptive coping mechanisms for the future. The intervention is time-limited, problem-focused, and oriented toward attainment of specific situationally appropriate goals. "The therapist should be skilled in rapid, accurate assessment of the patient's emotional status in recognition of both adaptive and maladaptive mechanisms, and in the immediate application of assessment information directly

related to the crisis in order to initiate effective intervention prevention, and early identification of emotional distress. (Capone et al., 1979)

How crisis affects the Mexican-American families and their extended families, and the mode of crisis intervention used with these families, will be the topic of this chapter. To fully understand the intricacies of the crisis, it is important to understand the Mexican-American family constellation. For this purpose, I will first describe the Mexican-American constellation, and then I will discuss the crisis and treatment phase.

THE MEXICAN-AMERICAN FAMILY

To make a definite statement describing the characteristics of the Mexican-American family is as difficult as trying to make one of the depolarized colors of the rainbow responsible for the nature of light. The present Mexican-Americans are as diverse as their cultural origin and historical heritage; from Indians, their conquerors, and the more recent prevalency of ethnic intermarriages. At present, it is not surprising to find Mexican-Americans with foreign middle or last names.

As a point of reference, I would like to refer to a border area on the Rio Grande neighboring the Mexican nation, Laredo, Texas. Before Laredo was founded, this area was inhabited by Indians—Apaches, Lepes—believed to have come either from the Pacific coast after crossing the Bering Strait, or from Mexico, as an expansion of the Aztec civilization. On May 15, 1755, Don Tomas Sanchez founded the province of Laredo. From then onward, Laredo underwent several political and governmental changes. Seven conquests took place, six flags went up, and six flags went down—Spanish, French, Mexican, Republic of the Rio Grande, Republic of Texas, and the Confederate Republic. The seventh flag, that of the United States, still flies, a result of the U.S. border crossing south over Laredo, rather than Laredo crossing north into the U.S. The transition (historical) under these different ruling nations, and the imposition of an anglo system and values on the people of Laredo as a result of the border moving south of Laredo, are factors which influence the characteristic make-up of the present Mexican-American generation. In my experience with Mexican-American families during 17 years in this area, I concur with the findings of Carolyn L. Attneave, who said in the book she coauthored with Ross V. Speck, *Family Networks* (1973), "I had lots of opportunity to observe many subcultures and to be aware not only of how similar people were, but also how many ways there were to arrange relationships."

It is safe to say, after studying the characteristics of the family, that throughout time families have remained basically about the same. It is also safe to assume that it is the necessities and the circumstances that change. In the existence of man, the necessities of a given time come at different cycles. However, the reactions to the necessities of life and the adjustment maneuvers are similar in their goals. The adjustment maneuvers may vary in accordance with the simplicity or sophistication of the people. The means used to reach the goal might be different, but the goal is about the same. The same can be said for family rearing in its variations and similarities.

We talk about Mexican-Americans, Mexicans of Hispanic descent without even realizing that we are excluding, to a great extent, important constitutive elements and in many instances a great deal of the elements are Indian ingredients. Those ingredients are also from a diverse cultural and historical background, comparable to the diversity of the cultural and historical roots of the Spanish conquerors who also underwent foreign domination—Arabian, Moors, Vikings, Gothic, Visigoth, and Ethiopians.

Stereotyping leads us to make big mistakes in evaluation, and with it, to have an even worse misunderstanding of any subject. Just for the sake of initiation, let us generalize first, and later see the subdivision of variance. Let us start with the schematic description of the Mexican-American family, speeding the evolution from the original Mexican family to the formation of a tribe as a convenient and life protecting organization. An organization needs to give power to a leader. The leader secured the assistance of his own family to govern the loyal subjects. Those subjects under this domination became dependent and submissive, with no self-determination or decision-making opportunities. The fathers of families under this form of government, had limited ownership of their children. They provided teaching the children their assigned roles. The Indian mother was very silent, and yet, very close to her children. But she was not too prone to externalize her feelings (feelings were secret), but the care and love were present. The Spanish domination (and the fall of the tribal form of government under the false promises of a different and better god) subjugated the families to the imposition of Spanish values. Either the Indians negated their own values or they faced death. Through 200 years of this domination, and the following 170 years of independence with a slow process of transitions in the Mexican Republic, and then through 138 years under the United States, the Mexicans and Mexican-American families have undergone a process of adjustment. That brings us to the present generation, where the old original characteristics and the new ones are accumulating, and where the exposures to new sets of values are now being confronted and accepted but not without internal or external conflicts.

Total Mexican-American Family

For the purpose of simplifying the understanding of the structure and functions of the Mexican-American family, I reviewed literature on what has been written and compiled regarding different characteristics of the Mexican-American families. I extracted those points where most authors have come into agreement, however with reservations, since there is not a significant amount of data compiled. With this in mind, and again with reservations, as a point of reference, I will describe the family as it has been stereotyped. This includes all the members of the family comparable to the modern nuclear family and all the extended members of that family. When we, as Mexicans or Mexican-Americans refer to my family, "mi familia," we consider all blood relatives as part of "mi familia." This does not mean the necessity for physical proximity of the family members, rather it means the existence of invisible, but strong and meaningful family ties. This pattern of family ties in the eyes of some Western civilizations has been insistently interpreted as overdependency, without considering that traditionally, and historically, the family as a total is a part of a twosome system of organization. The family is one system of organization and the surrounding world including the government and society is another. These are two separate systems. The system with the family in it has its own policies and society and its networks may have a different set of policies. In many instances where the policies differ, the family finds itself isolated from society.

For the sake of clarity, I will use the following nomenclature in relating to the family—"la familia": father and mother; son and daughter; paternal grandfather and paternal grandmother; maternal grandfather and maternal grandmother; uncles and aunts; uncle-in-law (tio politico) and aunt-in-law (tia politica), not blood related but related by marriage; and cousins (primos y primas).

Roles of The Family Members

Father. The father, from birth has gone through a progression of learning experiences already predesigned by the fact of his being male. In the early development process, even though his needs then are very similar to those of the baby girl, there still is a tinge of difference, especially in regards to exposing his body. This process gives grounds to imprinted values by the mere virtue of being male or female. As life proceeds, the direction given to the boy, as part of being male, is toward assuming the role of head of the household, a breadwinner later in life. In other words, the direction given is toward putting all his efforts into becoming a working person. The boy goes through the process of being very obedient, submissive, being told what to do and what to say in preparation to becoming the opposite on reaching adulthood. Adulthood, the legal voting age, and emotional maturity are not reached at the same time; the young man reaches maturity when he organizes his own family. Even then in his step toward a self-determined way of life, the ties with the original family are still not broken. The physical separation might be there; however, the emotional link persists and exists not as an imposition, but as a means of emotional support.

What has been described about the father's phases of development as a male, might be seen by some therapists as a rigid system. Thus, when evaluating his personality and behavior, the therapist could assume that male superiority is a doctrine that results in an authoritarian father. Carl E. Batt (1969), in his work *Mexican Character: An Adlerian Interpretation,* indicates that Samuel Ramos perceives Mexican in the Adlerian terms of inferiority complex, and the basic striving for security and superiority. Rogelio Diaz Guerrero (1955), states that the male presents problems of submission, conflict, and rebellion to authority; that he is preoccupied and anxious regarding his double role, when at times he must act maternally and tenderly, and at other times sexual and virile.

Mother. The mother, as female, seems to be more protected since birth. The indoctrination of being a woman, and her role as such, are initiated at an early age, begining with the types of toys she plays with, and soon after that, when some of the mother's chores are subtly introduced and then shared with the mother in preparation for motherhood. I do not know how much of this is conscious or unconscious participation. Girls are expected to be even more submissive than the boys. To accept dependency is feminine. Being delicate, discreet, is fostered and accepted by her own family as being feminine. After marriage, even though she lives within the same pattern and lifestyles, she assumes, or has to assume, a more directing, governing, and self-defined decision-making role. Paradoxically enough, this goes against what is generally assumed or believed. She becomes the nucleus, the strong pillar of the family, that intertwines all members of the family together. Still, there is a tendency to classify her as the submissive mother. From where does she get her strength? Undoubtedly, it may be attributed to the visible or invisible links and bonds still existing with her own family as a means of support. However, as Diaz Guerrero says:

> In the female, the main area of stress centers around her variable success in meeting the stiff requirements that culture demands [submission]. If she fails to meet her role expectation, self-belittlement and depressive trends are noted. Another area of

disturbance is found in the "old-maid" complex. With this in mind, we cannot wonder why, to some observers, when a father does not adopt the stereotype of the patriarchal style, or when a mother does not fulfill the expected pattern of a submissive wife, it is considered as deviance of psychopathology, or vice versa. Children basically go through the same process of development as their parents, with minimal changes that go along with the changes of society in any given time. Still, the persistence of obedience to the head of the family, and what is best for the family—passivity instead of assertiveness—continue to be emphasized.

With the passage of time, society changes. I am referring to the progress of civilization, by which the family, even the passive family, is influenced. Progress, such as the advancement of instant communication of events through the news media—radio, telephone, and television—if not completely convincing, is at least powerful enough to make an impact in reassessing values. Parents before us must have experienced the same impact as societal changes took place. There is no doubt that the news media and communication bombardments—under optimum circumstances—stimulate enrichment and progress. But in the Mexican-American families, the bombardment of information, which is at times opposite to cultural patterns, may provide grounds for conflicting evaluations and impeding or complicating an otherwise easy and painless decision-making process and may cause contradictory emotional battles over having to restrain the new acquired goals that oppose those of the parents.

The Extended Family

The extended family is a strong support system and provides not only warmth, but also protection against breakdown, and will provide continued support should a breakdown occur.

The Grandparents.   Most of these elderly persons, or a great majority of them, are not only Mexican descendants, but in many instances have come from Mexican villages, rather than from cities. While in the United States, they have to face cultures totally foreign to theirs. In their attempt to acculturate, or to organize themselves, they experience a difficult and painstaking process. Then they usually remain as they were with all their patterns unchanged. However, their continued importance within the family, which of course pleases them, is still evident and they seem to be in their element in the homes. They remain relatively unacculturated, preserving the traditional Mexican pattern to a great extent (Clark and Mendelson, 1969).

Grandparents, as was previously mentioned, still exercise some influence on their grandchildren. This influence is meaningful not only by their physical presence and emotional support, but also as a memory chest of old values—cultural, historical, emotional. The consistency of these values have built the columns of a building housing security as a savings deposit to count on in time of need.

Placing grandparents in long-term institutions—hospitals, nursing homes—because of illness or age is very seldom seen. If it must be done, it is not without emotional conflict. Grandparents are usually kept at home, and this has proved to be less detrimental to the emotional and physical well-being of the elderly.

Aunts and Uncles. Aunts and uncles contribute a great deal during the lifetime of the family. They contribute as providers of extended parenthood to their nieces and nephews and are seen by the niece and nephew with the same respect and obedience they give their own parents.

Cousins. Cousins usually, because of physical (residential) proximity, become natural playmates giving each other protection and peer supervision. The younger learn from the older.

RELATIONSHIPS

First, I will elaborate on the interrelationship among members of the family network and their two-way influence on family members, and then I will discuss the external family network ramifications.

The influence exerted by the grandparents will depend upon the parents chronological position in the family, and their sex, a distinction that is tolerated because it has been indoctrinated in such a way that it has become an acceptable pattern.

We note that after marriage the child's spouse is included in the family circle, but not without some adaptation. The spouse is added on to the new family while remaining in the other family. The grandfathers, in an unwritten agreement, are granted a certain amount of participation in family matters as an expected moral and emotional obligation on their part.

The father's siblings are also influenced by the established pattern of the grandparents and through their proximity and togetherness share the influence on the father. They reach out for each other for mutual support and interaction.

Mutual influence is exerted by cousins—male and female—in their world of a child. They are usually about the same age and become mutual first playmates. In relating to cousins of both sexes, the child learns to get along with others and is exposed to both sexes and learns about the differences in sexes and sex roles. This interaction enhances the individual's knowledge and understanding and prepares him/her for the time when he/she makes the choice of a spouse and starts his/her own family—a continuation of the one he/she came from.

Whether the family is to survive and face conflicts depends upon how the external ramifications may affect the close-knit family network. In many instances, the confrontation with opposing sets of societal values (as happens with the Mexican-Americans in the United States) is the precipitating factor of a crisis. The close-knit family network does not exclude inner interpersonal conflict caused by the members' individual idiosyncracies. There is a family tendency to try to resolve these conflicts themselves. We say: "la ropa sucia se lava en casa," which means, "the dirty linen is washed at home," or in other words, "keep the family skeletons in the closet."

I will enumerate some of the most widely known ramifications, since in every area people will seek those ramifications or relationships they can establish in accordance with the available resources of the area—midwife, curandero(a), etc.

Compadres

One of the family's first chosen relationships is the selection of a compadre-comadre (godfather-godmother). The godparent will represent for the child an extension of the parents in case of the parents absence because of illness, death, etc. It is not necessarily a legal responsibility, but it does represent a moral responsibility. This is why their choice is a meticulous one, and why the chosen one(s) feel privileged at having been chosen and given that honor and trust. The compadres of christening or baptism are first in priority, in importance, and in close relationship to the family. Then come the compadres of confirmation and marriage.

Friends

Friends are not actually chosen, but rather are the result of the circumstance of togetherness because of physical proximity in school or neighborhood. During school days, groups are formed or selected and children spend many hours each day interacting and consequently forming friendships.

Doctors

Mexican-Americans are selective in choosing a doctor because of their belief in the sanctity of the human body and modesty of exposing themselves, especially the female. This might explain the still prevalent use of midwives—not only because of economics, but because husbands feel very sensitive about their wives being touched by another man. Once they find their family doctor, easier nowadays because of women physicians, they keep this doctor practically for life. Many times the doctor's services are sought for more than health care, such as advice on marriage problems, educational difficulties, behavioral problems, etc.

Folk Medicine

In certain segments of the population, there is the alternative to medical doctors—the use of the curanderismo, faith healers, spiritualists, palm readers, card readers, and herbal medicine dealers; all are referred to as folk medicine. Curanderismo is the art of healing. It has existed long before conventional medical care, and has always been a resource used by Mexican-Americans. Curanderismo has been traced to ancient Indian civilizations, with many elements brought over from the Old World by the conquerors. The reason for its use represents the most meaningful, effective, and economical means of relief from physical and psychological illness. It is also pertinent to mention that Mexican-Americans feel that, while conventional health care is capable of healing physical ailments, it does not meet their psychological needs.

The authentic curandero, even though many may be "quacks," has rigid professional ethics, extensive healing knowledge, and a strong devotion for his work. Curanderos who have a good reputation are the only ones who survive, and almost never have a set fee for services. They appear to be motivated toward helping people rather than making money. "Payment," they usually say, "I leave it to your conscience." They see their work as a spiritual vocation rather than as a business enterprise; to heal is a gift of God. They emphasize that the patient's faith aids the healing process. The curandero is very capable of establishing a close relationship with the patient, instilling confidence and helping them to overcome their fears. Some curanderos read medical books as well as psychiatric books, and when the case needs a doctor's intervention, it is referred to the doctor. However, since their profession is seen with skepticism by doctors, doctors do not refer patients to curanderos.

Teachers

Children are more or less indoctrinated to see the teacher as a second mother. Teachers have an intense influence on the child, so the interaction between teacher and pupil, especially female teacher and pupil, is a sort of continuation of the mother–child relationship. The child's behavior as observed in school may be the basis for the teacher to form an idea of the home situation. Perhaps a study or research project should be made into the relationship and interaction between the younger aged child and the male and female teachers in a day-care and kindergarten environment. This is the age where valuable information could be obtained for early intervention and prevention of later developmental disturbances. The teacher could be a good resource, not only in obtaining information, but also because of her/his importance in the child's life, the teacher could provide beneficial intervention in a conjoint helping process.

Religion

Religion has been a strong support system for all humanity and especially so for Mexican-Americans. Because of its form of indoctrination, it is not only a supportive system but a disciplinary, punitive, and also guilt-ridden system. It was imposed forcefully (historically) and resulted in submission, fatalism, or in the hope for a better life after death. Because of all this, Mexican-Americans see the representative of the church as the ruling judge of rightness or wrongness in their life, an advisor, and at times, when the occasion presents itself, a dispenser of lenient punishment. So the people are not afraid of the priest, instead, they trust him more than they trust their parents.

Neighbors

The characteristics of the neighborhood members are somewhat like isolated islands. Each island has its own private lifestyle. There is a tendency to unite but mostly in times of catastrophe rather than in times of private affairs or festivities. This is sort of an unwritten contract, and when incidents happen and help is needed, neighbors readily and voluntarily give it, not offer it. If we, the therapists, need to turn to neighbors for assistance, it has to be done with tact and the knowledge that the family in stress has the right of privacy and only the family can evaluate if it is the right time for the neighbors to participate.

There are other relationships that a family might have which are too lengthy to be explained because of the specificity of each family. These relationships should be investigated or evaluated for future planning in resource utilization.

CRISIS IN MEXICAN-AMERICAN FAMILIES

Crisis is an emotionally significant event or radical change of status in a person's life. The life is disrupted from its usual mode of adaptation. The events or radical changes of status that can affect the Mexican-American families and their extended families can be divided into two categories: inner family conflicts, and family conflicts caused when confronting external influences.

Inner family conflicts may arise from the loss of the head of the household (breadwinner), or of an important family member owing to death, desertion, abandonment, separation, retirement, or to the incapacitation of the head of the household because of prolonged illness, disability, or old age. Included here also are those family interrelationships affected negatively by influences outside of the family unit, and by some members, or member, whose behavior, being foreign to the family, might cause a break in the previous homeostasis of the family. It is these outside influences that to a great extent, disrupt the harmony of the family, while some of their members in their struggle for "acculturation and assimilation" into the overpowering society cause conflict.

Figure 8–1 graphically shows the surrounding elements in which the family exists and navigates, in which mutual configurations definitely affect the family positively or negatively. The cones shown in the figure indicate the acceptance, or inclusion into the family of those elements favorable to them, while the others are most likely to be questionable, unacceptable, and stress-provoking elements. All the elements mentioned in Figure 8–1 form that part of the outside society in which the family exists.

Despite historical facts that the United States was founded on the principle of equality among people, an abundance of data exists to indicate that this great society has held and still continues to hold, a series of discriminatory attitudes toward various ethnic, racial, and cultural groups. Prejudice is a maintained belief by a large segment of the dominant society that the Spanish-speaking population, for example Mexican-Americans, possess a pattern of negatively valued traits. People tend to perceive "differences" (they are different from us now, consequently, they are negative and unfavorable) (Padilla and Ruiz, 1976).

An individual or a family can find serious problems when he/they try to adapt to the social mores of an alien culture. Interaction with the representatives of social systems can strongly affect the individual's or family's self-esteem (Cohen, 1970).

Mexican-Americans are in many instances exposed to a hostile and excluding attitude, to multiple detrimental conditions conducive to a psychosocial dysfunction and psychiatric impairment. Yet, as is typically the case with the Spanish-speaking population (Mexican-American), in spite of the level of need, services are underutilized. Within this exposure to the external society, or in reference to the external world

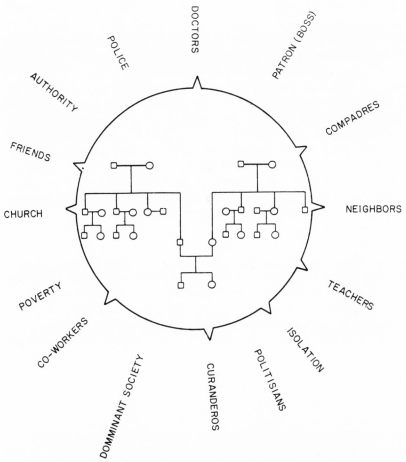

DOCTORS

POLICE

PATRON (BOSS)

AUTHORITY

COMPADRES

FRIENDS

CHURCH

NEIGHBORS

POVERTY

TEACHERS

CO-WORKERS

ISOLATION

POLITISIANS

DOMMINANT SOCIETY

CURANDEROS

**Figure 8–1.   Social Network, Total Social Matrix, Social
Support System, Retribalization.**

of the family, stress-producing elements could be mainly attributed to the confrontation with different sets of values.

Conflicting cultural norms complicate acculturation. To what extent do the Mexican-American values conflict with the American values? How are such cultural conflicts resolved—individually or by the family? It is a fact that the roots of the language are challenged, modified, or in need of replacement in the resocialization process into the American way of life. The change of the interpersonal relationships and cultural norms, the absence of verbal aggression, direct expression of one's own feelings, and the avoidance of confrontation, are personal qualities that are highly esteemed personal virtues. Competition is conflicting with their own pattern. The lack of assertiveness, is interpreted about the Mexican-American as shameful. The reaching of ideal goals is more important to the family than the individual. Family name or honor is reinforced by the rule of not discussing problems outside of the family. When all these factors are confronted with a different dominant society, it definitely gives room for a closed conflict, and from conflict develops stress (Sook and Toupin, 1980).

Another exposure to the external conflict-producing elements is the dependency of the family on the secure subsistence provided by the employer. In the area where the vast majority of families depend upon the productivity of the seasonal harvest, these families are exposed to the viscissitudes of nature, drought, fire, frost, etc., and currently an ever-growing farming technology which decreases employment opportunities for manual laborers. Their lack of other employment skills gives grounds for stress and for an uncertain future.

External authority differs from internal family authority, creating conflicts within the family members in relation to discipline and civil rights. The conflicting impact of the public education system versus family education creates, not only a wider generation gap, but an inner overwhelming conflict in which the bombardment comes from two opposing and contradictory set of values—the individual values of the dominant society on one side versus the family traditional values on the other. In many instances this provides the stage on which parents and children cannot communicate in a common language, which in a very sensitive manner will or may lead to, not only the physical gap, but the emotional separation that disrupts the interdependency of the family members, with the consequential stress-producing effects.

It is also within this area of discussion where the evaluation of the person's performance is misinterpreted by some, and many characteristics are considered as deviant instead of culturally normal. With this in mind, this sector of the Mexican-American population is excluded from certain benefits that they could share with other segments of society. This lack of future expectations on the part of Mexican-Americans, for security and progress contributes to disenchantment, and a fatalistic, pessimistic and anxiety producing frustration.

Police harassment has been frequently reported, not only toward Mexican-Americans, but toward other minorities as well. Perhaps harassment has gone to extremes because of preconceived expectations of the authorities toward the minorities. Thus, the minorities fulfill the prophecy of the role already assigned to them with the expectation that, in spite of all the deprivation the minorities have experienced, their behavior should be better than that exhibited by the members of the dominant society. This reminds me of an old Mexican saying in reference to exuberant expressions of emotions and behavior, "lo del pobre es borrachera, y lo del rico es alegria," "in the poor it is drunkenness, in the rich it is happiness."

> In all, it is very clearly manifested, that the Mexican-American family tends to come into conflict with the dominant society because the value system contrasts sharply with that of the minority, and because no substantial effort has been made to adapt services to the basic difference in consequent diverging needs. (Saenz, 1978)

Broad physical, psychological, social, and family changes have a powerful impact on members of the family. The members are compelled to adjust, not only to rapid individual changes, but also to meet simultaneously, the expectations of both—family and community. Stress is to be expected, but for some, it might become overwhelming. As in the psychological sphere, any disturbance in the homeostasis between man and his surroundings is also translated into a disturbance of the intellect's emotional or behavioral spheres, separately or together. It is our obligation to become custodians of the homeostasis, preventing the nature of the surrounding elements from continuing to change in search of the obsessive flourishing of a dehumanizing technology. Man is adaptable, yes, but also deformable.

Crisis Intervention

Crisis intervention in psychotherapy is often a harrowing experience for both patient (family) and therapist. The intensity and immediacy of an individual family in torment and anguish can shatter the most effective and serene therapeutic relationship. The appeal to reason and reality is often impotent with someone who experiences his world tumbling down around him (them). The usual code of behavior between therapists and patients is no longer operative, and there is a need for a fast, practical, concrete response to the situation. Such an experience can be an opportunity for the therapist to employ his creativity in utilizing untapped resources to help cope with this crisis. This creativity might be the one that can trace the route, and outline the steps to follow in an attempt to accommodate the diversity of specific needs to specific families. Too intense plans could be primarily contemplated in dealing with the Mexican-American family, extended family, and its surroundings (total social matrix), in an attempt to initiate the evaluation of the situation in whichever way it might be more accessible and feasible. Let us say that in Figure 8–1 we go from the periphery of the diagram to the center (family) or from the center (family) to the periphery. As it has already been said, with the family having such a strict code of secrecy, the therapist must proceed tactfully with respect to the family's reluctance in seeking help, because in some instances, it may connote change or shamefulness of being mentally sick or in need of help. It is very important, to keep in mind that the involvement with the family is most comfortable and powerfully accomplished through sincere and well-intentioned maneuvers. The primary difficulty is that the family members seek help in an incomplete condition, that is, after the damage has been done. They do not seem to have the healing energy they previously had. We need a clear idea about how the disrupted family or the family in crisis works, and what can be done to help it. A very widespread misbelief among orthodox psychiatrists or psychoanalysts is that when these families (remnants) are approached, they are quite resistant to change (Peck, 1975).

The fact remains that the practitioners of these procedures have neglected, or seem to neglect, that in analysis all ingredients should be analyzed—not just those that fit our elaborated maps or scripts. When our scripts are narrow, our analysis is narrow. We need to widen our scripts, by including new ingredients, so that we can have a clear idea of the analysant, in this case the Mexican-American family, how it works and what can be done at the pace the emergency requires, and not just giving a band-aid treatment because of their unsuitability for analysis. For this reason I feel that we have to help the providers to clarify their understanding, hopefully stirring up their own biases and feelings which prevent them from their own involvement. Involvement is accomplished more comfortably and powerfully when a sincere and well-intentioned commitment is achieved.

A primary difficulty for the family's sake is that by the time the family seeks outside help, damage has already been done, "palo dado ni Dios lo quita." As we say in Spanish, "once hit with a stick, not even God can take it away," or "for damage done, nothing can be undone." However, this does not exclude our responsibility of preventing new occurrences. One of the most paradoxical things is that many Mexican-Americans are going through more than their share of the unpleasantness of life. They have suffered throughout history with poverty, being unskilled, unemployed, having a high percentage of school dropouts, lacking political representation, poor health, poor housing, lacking mastery of the English language, bilingualism (that instead of being recognized as an achievement is considered as a handicap for progress), prolific families (interpreted as too many for so little, in relation to care and love), discrimination, the handicapping roles of male and female (male stereotyped as "macho," meaning abusive, irresponsible, pleasure seeker, etc.; and the female as a submissive, dependent, worth nothing more than for childrearing and being a built-in housekeeper. These situations in a so-called normal socially accepted patterned family would precipitate a mental breakdown). However, research data reflect the underutilization of mental health services by Mexican-Americans, who according to some, are the ones that need it most. This makes us wonder whether the Mexican-Americans are more immune to the stress which cause emotional or mental disorders or if the emotional disorders are hidden, untreated, and handled in some other way which avoids the use of mental health services. Or could it be that the mental health services are inadequate, unreliable, obsolete, inaccessible, and irrelevant to the needs of the Mexican-American? Is it possible that the staff of the services have personal characteristics and attitudes which do not allow the establishment of rapport because of preconceived and mutual stereotyping. Bringing Mexican-Americans into the mainstream of mental health is an arduous task requiring more than initial effort. Rather, it may require long-term commitment in a variety of methods or approaches, perhaps something more informal and nonthreatening. Most important, even before any elaborated program or plan is drawn, professionals should not,only learn how to approach the Mexican-Americans but also how to be accepted by them, hoping that this will ease future negotiations and the establishment of a trust and comaradry facilitating a therapeutic relationship. This is especially important for those who do not seek mental health care but are either referred, forced to come, or strongly advised to seek help because of being found by the sender as "deviant."

In working with the Mexican-American family and extended family, I have found that there is not only a very strong support system within the family, but within the chosen external members of the society as well. The chosen external members offer a mutual help system that prevents the family from going to the "traditional therapeutic system." This mutual help system consists of the mutuality and reciprocity in need satisfaction. Each time an individual (family unit) or the prolongation of the family (social matrix) in which the family lives, gives control and nurtures another family member, the action benefits the giver as much and sometimes more than the recipient. Helping activity within the family circle may involve sublimated elements of altruism, but the importance of self-interest is not hard to identify. A parent has a basic urge to nurture and profits from satisfying this drive, just as much as each child may benefit from being guided, supported, and loved.

By breaking down the components between family members, it becomes possible to see how factors such as power, closeness, problem solving dealt with, will affect the lives and families. It is also possible to see how these factors can be used in understanding the family, and in working toward finding alternatives in helping when the human strengths holding the families together, have broken down.

As the younger generation attempts to acculturate and become a part of their peer group, they adopt some of the values which will be in conflict with the family values. In many instances this represents a threat to the stability and unity of the family constellation. This can precipitate a crisis in which the therapist may become involved, not only as a therapist, but as a judge of the rightness or wrongness of the family members. Being a judge is a role I have always tried to avoid. I have found it is very effective to bring all the family members together as well as important persons in their own social network, young and old, and under my mediation discuss the matter in their diverse perspectives or points of view. A typical example of this is when the youngsters learn, through their relationship with their peers the rights acquired when they reach eighteen—the age at which certain privileges have been granted to others, but are unseen and unacceptable to his family unit. It is through a long process of discussion of the parents' fear, mistrust, disgust, anxiety, and of the youngsters' rebellion, or dissatisfaction on what they consider extremely imposed discipline, that the whole family may reach a happy medium, with certain concessions as well as obligations being reached. All these add up with the preservation of some of the parental values with the addition of moderate changes, but based on the youngsters' making themselves trustworthy and for the elders to stand the waiting.

Facing the crisis of the loss of the breadwinner by death, for instance, the family network and the social network usually immediately will try to take care of this crisis, even if they were not prepared for it. They pull their resources together to take care of the immediate situation. Since extreme emotional display in mourning is an expected reaction, family members, or those in the social network, do not discourage this channelization of emotions. They, at times, even encourage, in a supportive manner, the mourners to cry. This has the benefits of the catharsis. Thus, depression does not usually appear at this time. The need for intervention by the therapist at this time is almost impractical or inadvisable. It is not only impractical, but ineffective and not recommended, since it prevents the individual from manifesting spontaneous feelings with the result of more damaging flashbacks. With certain variations, the loss of a person is handled by the conjoint effort of the family, but the delegation of responsibilities may be voluntarily undertaken by a family member. This family member will be the person that might very likely, if not ready, suffer the overwhelming responsibility resulting in a conflict. It would be until then that he/she might be referred, or that he/she might feel the need for help. But he/she cannot express this conflict within the family, but he/she might look for outside help, incapable of accepting the guilt of what he/she considers his/her failure before the family. This may sound as though the psychotherapist does not have a place or function within this network. Apparently the family is very well equipped to deal with the situation. However, this is ideally conceived when the family has the means and ways to do it—financially, or as a group, in numbers and possibilities and participation. But when the whole family is conflicting with the dominant society, when in its transactions the family gets a smaller piece of the pie, and when the strengths of the family are weakened, cut off, broken down, etc., because of the overwhelming conflict, the psychotherapist can, as knowledgeable person of both systems, moderate and stimulate the family toward a more mutually satisfying situation based on the strengths of both, instead of on the strengths of one versus the weaknesses of the other (Lewis, 1979).

I have found that families are inner-directed and typically will shun outside care. In many instances, they will try to rely on their own resources (Caplan and Killilea, 1976) and those of their own close friends and associates. For a family used to supporting (intracultural) help practices for generations, there has to be a promise of an important pay-off if it is to try a new system.

There is a strong attachment to the extended family which also functions as a natural resource and support system even in adulthood. While faith healers and curanderos(as) appear to be diminishing in number, they are still easily accessible, inexpensive, and adapted to the culture of the barrio. They are respectful of the old family traditions. They have credibility (Clark, 1969).

With this in mind, instead of discarding this as superstition, fanaticism, or something not acceptable by the professional scientific world, do not condemn the family for using either or both of these systems, because families many times are aware that they can have conventional health care capable of healing physical ailments, but that this does not meet their psychological needs fulfilled by the confidence of the curanderos(as). The same goes for all the empirical maneuvers and practices that the family has been utilizing traditionally from generation to generation, which successfully provides healing elements by the mutual supporting help provided in their own capacity by mutual members of the nuclear family, extended family, and the social network integrated into the family.

I see forthcoming the flourishing of the family network therapy, and the networks around it, aware and very convinced, that the therapy could not be possible without the tremendous, powerful impact, importance, and healing qualities of the family members and their network. I am indebted to family therapists: Ackerman, Caplan, Speck, Attneave, Whittaker, Satir, Shwartz, Serrano, and other important contributors, but more so to those directly responsible for the healing, the members of the families, in my case the Mexican-American families and extended families. As for myself, I am greatly indebted, not only by being a descendant of a Mexican family, cradle of myself, but for what my people have taught me in my association with them.

VIGNETTES

1. Ramon, his wife Maria, and their six children (Juanita, Pedro, Pablo, Chucho, Jacinto, and Jose) every year in the early spring, packed their belongings to go up north to harvest, as he, his extended family, and others like him have been doing from generation to generation. Life went by rather smoothly with only everyday problems which were not too hard to be solved. With the years the parents and children were growing older, the trips began to be more of an effort for Ramon, and the expenses increased as the children grew older. One summer while on their annual journey, to their misfortune, they found out that the harvesting had been mechanized, and there was no job for Ramon and the family. They spent that season doing whatever jobs came along just to survive and to meet the expenses of the trip. They returned home as a depressed family. The members began to look for work in town, but owing to their lack of skills, they found it difficult to find a job they could perform. Ramon, who was a very proud Mexican, found it shameful to ask for assistance. The children did not want to remain in school, with the consequent chain reaction within the school system attempting to keep the children in school. The school staff initiated legal proceedings against the parents. Ramon, who had never been a disrespectful person, proud of his family and had lived a happy and private life until now, under the pressures from the school and from the lack of an opportunity to make a living, reached the point of frustration and protested and rebelled against the school's action, saying that he had reared a nice family, had never gotten into trouble, and had taught his children and would keep on teaching them the way he wanted. He went to the extreme of threatening, saying that if they kept pushing him around, he was going to do some harm to whoever showed up at his house to take the children. This is why the family was referred to me. In a delicate situation like this, the therapist, for his own protection, has to seek the available resources in the best and safe way to attempt to reach the family. In other words, what was mentioned before about moving from the periphery of the structure to the center was the method used by me. So a network was established, consisting of visiting teachers, truant officers, and counselors, who

searched for the important people around the identified problem family in crisis. Their search was not obvious because they were people who usually visited and mingled with the neighborhood. They were able to elicit through normal conversations who were the important people to the family. It is not something one can rush into. One has to take the attitude that the surgeon takes in the incision of a boil, wait till the time is right. Through many informal conversations, PTA meetings, and in a very subtle manner, general situations were discussed so the neighborhood families could get the hint that there were many problems in school and that dropouts were not such a unique happening. The idea was that the dropout situation could only be alleviated with the parents' participation in the education of the child. In the network's efforts to motivate them, they explained the benefits of education versus noneducation. The PTA group decided to search for ways of helping the children with their education, such as tutoring. Through the PTA group, parents who knew the family with the problem (Ramon and his family), in neighborly conversations conveyed the idea of tutoring the children, and help was provided by this group. The children returned to school and I never saw the family.

2.   Francisco is a merchant who came as a young child from a town in Mexico in a horse-drawn cart whose driver offered him a ride. He came in search of a job. He found a job as a messenger and cleaning boy in a general mercantile store. In a few months he learned the trade and was promoted to behind-the-counter sales clerk. As he grew older, persistence and tenacity made him decide to organize a partnership and establish his own store. He got married, had children, and educated them. At the same time his business was prospering and becoming an important store in the area. As years went by and he was already well established, the children who were grown, were on their own and prosperous too, saw that he was behind in the modern ways of transaction, even though he was profiting, however not as they thought he should. They decided to implement some changes to modernize the business—changes that the father very vehemently rejected with his own philosophy of the traditional self-made man—"I did well without modern technology. I educated you well." The family, together, in the assumption that they had to do the right thing, asked for my participation in dealing with the stubborn old man. The wife was very much convinced by her children that what they were doing was in the best interest of the father, who, they felt, was making too many demands on his own person—overworking, becoming easily upset, stubborn, etc., and sometimes they felt he was preventing the store from growing more. The family arranged a meeting for me to meet with the parents in an informal meeting with the excuse that they wanted me to see the mother, who, being a diabetic, was experiencing depressive episodes.

My plan was to meet them and make an evaluation of the characteristics of the parents' personalities, and then to arrange for other visits to meet with the rest of the family for an overview of the family situation. It was not difficult for me to establish a good relationship with the parents, even though the man expressed the fact that he wondered if one of his sons had sent me to check on him, and he said to me about his son that, "he may have read a lot, but he does not know anything." In reference to that, I said that his son worried about him and did not want anything to happen to him. After that we established a positive rapport on a casual, but productive exchange of ideas on life, life situations, etc., which made him feel that he could trust me, since I was the only one he could communicate with, without being critical. I held separate family meetings with the rest of the family members, including the grandchildren and the in-laws. After evaluation, confrontations, and reevaluations, the children became more receptive about the needs of the father and found an alternative solution, benefitting both children and parents, mainly through the change of attitude developed in the meeting sessions. They themselves, without my physical presence, settled the conflict with an even more profitable solution than was previously proposed.

3.   A very hardworking businessman, Federico Sr., was a very righteous, precise, methodic, demanding European immigrant who came seeking for a varied way of life and through hard work, managed to own a store, and married a typical Mexican-American girl in those times—submissive, nonopinionated, passive—who needed a strong character to lean on. They had two sons and two daughters, and some members of her family lived in her house. The four children became professionals and very prominent in their own fields. The father always had the idea that at least one of his children would follow his steps to maintain the love of his life, the store, where he had spent most of his time to build it up. Under his guidance and strong direction the family was very united and always did things together. The first encounter with unhappiness was when the children began to leave town in pursuit of their education. The second was when the father found out that none of the children were interested in the store. The third was when one of the children decided to marry and the father saw this as the beginning of the family break-up, especially due to the fact that it was the oldest who wanted to marry. Since he was more or less the head of the house while his father was dedicated mainly to the store, it disrupted the family to the extreme that the youngest daughter had a breakdown, and at this point the case was referred to me. I initiated treatment with the identified patient, continuing with family therapy, and then extending to the extended family, then extending to friends of the siblings. Through the process of these sessions became apparent the effect of separations on all members of the family, transmitted

from the father's reaction to separation of his own place of origin and the extreme defensive maneuvers he utilized to obtain the security that he could only find in the business and in his own family's symbiosis, as if the separation was going to be forever and as such, hazardous and painful. Through the sessions and reevaluation of the anxiety in the mutual self-help there was provided a more objective and realistic expectation of each other. With this family there have been other episodes of crisis, but my participation in the intervention has not been as lengthy as it was before.

Conclusion

Crisis intervention in the Mexican-American family, even though in many instances should be handled as any other family crisis intervention in any ethnic group, has its variable due to the family constellation which includes the nuclear family, extended family, and the adopted external relationships in a homeostatic interaction and living in continued interdependency on one hand, and on the other hand, the external world foreign to the ways of life and seen as threatening to the homeostatic balance of the family. It is of extreme importance to underline the mutual aspects of all the support systems of mutuality and reciprocity (Caplan and Killilea, 1976). Our participation as therapists is to facilitate the continuation of the strengths (Caplan, 1972) that this unity has and for these families to achieve unity in such a way that they become confident enough, strong enough, assertive enough, not as individuals, but as a family or as a group, in their immediate network and the external society. Once this is attained, they can negotiate with the upsetting stressful factors, those that are provoked by the overpowering dominant society, who, in turn, will be more capable of elaborating plans, programs, help, health-care systems, etc., relevant to the needs specific to this segment, based on the nature of the needs expressed by this group. Perhaps the role of the psychotherapist is to stir up the situation so all the elements will come to the surface and become easily recognizable, stimulating all the members at their own pace and capacity to the resolution of the problem by eliminating the damaging elements and increasing the ones that might produce benefit. Sensibility of the therapist is a quality, not a learning experience. So those who have it will not find it difficult to understand and help. Those who do not, will expose society to the same damaging impact that the dominant influence and stressful elements are producing—the conflict—by their obsessive, well-intentioned desire for innovative change, as has been mentioned before. In closing, it is our obligation to become the custodians of the homeostasis beginning through the family toward society in general, preventing the nature of all the elements from continuing to damage in the search of the obsessive flourishing of a dehumanizing technology, keeping in mind that man is adaptable, yes, but he is deformable too.

REFERENCES

Amada, G. Crisis-oriented psychotherapy: Some theoretical and practical considerations. *Journal of Contemporary Psychotherapy,* 1977, *9*(1).

Batt, C. E. Mexican character: An Adlerian interpretation. *Journal of Individual Psychology,* 1969.

Caplan, G. *Support system and community mental health on concept development.* New York: Human Sciences Press, 1974.

Caplan, G. and Killilea, M. *Support systems and mutual help: Multidisciplinary explorations.* New York: Grune and Stratton, 1976.

Capone, M. A., Westie, K. S., Chitwood, J., Fiegenbaum, D., and Good, R. S. Crisis intervention: A functional model for hospitalized cancer patients. *American Journal of Orthopsychiatry,* 1979, *49*(1), 598–607.

Clark, M. and Mendelson, M. Mexican-American aged in San Francisco: A case description. *Gerontology,* 1969, *9.*

Cohen, R. E. Preventive mental health programs for ethnic minority population: A case in point. Paper presented at the Congresso Internacional de Americanistas Lima, Peru, 1970 (mimeo).

Diaz Guerrero, R. Neurosis and the Mexican family structure. *American Journal of Psychiatry,* 1955, *112*(6).

Group for the Advancement of Psychiatry. *Mental retardation: A family crisis.* Report No. 56, December, 1963.

Healthy people: The Surgeon General's report on health promotion and disease control. United States Department of Health, Education and Welfare, Pub. No. 79-55071, Washington: 1969.

Lewis, J. N. *How is your family? A guide to identifying your family's strengths and weaknesses.* New York: Brunner/Mazel, 1979.

Padilla, A. and Ruiz, R. *Latino mental health.* United States Department of Health, Education and Welfare. Bethesda, Md.: NIMH, 1976.

Peck, B. B. Psychotherapy with disrupted families. *Journal of Contemporary Psychotherapy,* 1975, *7.*

Saenz, J. The value of a humanistic model in serving families. *Hispanic Families.* COSSMHO, 1978.

Slide Series. *Curanderismo: An optional health care system.* Pan American University, 1975.

Sook, E. and Toupin, W. Counseling Chinese Asians: Psychotherapy in the context of racism and Asian-American history. *American Journal of Orthopsychiatry,* 1980, *50*(1), 76–86.

Speck, R. V. and Attneave, C. L. *Family networks.* New York: Pantheon Books, 1973.

Chapter 9

JUVENILE DELINQUENCY AND FAMILY SYSTEMS

Thomas F. Johnson, Ph.D.

The arguments for a family systems and family therapy approach to juvenile delinquency are explored in this chapter by Thomas Johnson. Traditionally the problem has been seen as either in the personality of the delinquent or in the social forces in which he/she grew up. Treatment has frequently been handed to the judiciary. This chapter stresses that the problem lies in the family system and treatment is most effective if this is the unit of therapy.

THE DELINQUENT AS PARTICIPANT

It is human nature to structure problems as either-or situations. There is something very compelling about such propositions. The common wisdom is filled with such constructions and we all tend to fall in with them.

One of the first departures from polarity to be made has to do with the question: "Who is the victim?" The answer might properly be that everyone is the victim and no one is the victim. The idea that there is a victim is closely tied to the idea that the realm being considered is essentially a dichotomy. Without an either-or structure, the usefulness of determining who is victim diminishes and may lose meaning altogether.

A more fruitful and more realistic view would be to consider the juvenile delinquent as a participant in the events of his own life. It is true that human beings are subject to many forces over which there is little if any possibility for control. But the manner in which the individual goes about life may not only modify the impact of the forces which affect him, but may set forces in motion as well. Our relationships with other people have much to do with what we do and what we become. These relationships profoundly influence the way in which we live our lives. There appear to be certain patterns of response that endure. There is what Jackson has called a redundancy to behavior, patterns which occur over and over in regular sequences (Jackson, 1957). It is these enduring patterns which justify the use of a concept such as "personality" to identify and describe a given individual. Entrenched and resistant to change as these patterns may be, it is also evident that there are certain situations which elicit different patterns. These are patterns, already part of the individual's repertoire, but not often used. They are there, available when changing circumstances call for them. They become apparent in different contexts and often are referred to as role-playing. These acts are attempts to work out a relationship with others in the situation. They are not static but involve changes, many of them subtle and unrecognized, as well as unacknowledged. They represent adjustments which will eventually establish the relationships of those participating in the situation. As Shibutani (1961), the sociologist, noted:

> The direction taken by a person's conduct is seen as something that is constructed in the reciprocal give and take of interdependent men who are adjusting to one another.

The reciprocal nature of a response implies interpersonal contexts for behavior and may be understood as universal. Within a given context, all parties are by definition participant. There are no bystanders, inasmuch as standing by is a way of functioning in a particular situation, with consequences for everyone present. Those who are identified as actors must necessarily be operating not only by taking account of the other active persons, but also by taking account of those who are being inactive. In the same way, a youngster engaged in some act of delinquency is a participant. He is not merely engaged with a friend in performing an act that will establish his credentials, such as the new boy taking a dare, or an outsider wanting to become part of the in group. Nor is there necessarily anything at stake with respect to the victim of the delinquency. Both possibilities may exist as themes and their existence may appear to give them the status of major aspects. Convention bids us look at events in this way: the aggressor and the victim are clearly visible. Everyone can agree readily to participation of this sort. What is more difficult, is to find and recognize another order of participation: participation in the maintaining of a social system.

THE FAMILY AS A SOCIAL SYSTEM

Human beings function within social systems which operate at many levels. Each system is characterized by being organized by means of a set of rules. The rules make it possible for the system to function since the interaction between members is governed by them. As is the case for all social systems, "the family is a rule-governed system" (Jackson, 1957). Within the family system, each member is engaged in reciprocal interaction with the others. When the give and take of these relationships leads to agreement, the effect is a contribution to the stability of the system. When agreement cannot be reached, an instability results which prompts corrective measures. Until the correction succeeds, the family system will be disrupted and may ultimately be destroyed. The fact that the central dynamic is agreement among the members allows for flexibility. The possibility of renegotiating and modifying the rules is implied and in this way, through reopening established principles it is possible to meet new exigencies. Reassessment and modification are ongoing features of a family system. Internal and external changes are a constant of life. As they occur, the impact upon family members will make readjustments necessary.

At any given point it may be difficult for the family to agree upon the rules which govern the system and whatever has changed or threatens to change may create a strain for a long period of time. Father may have been defined as head of the household, but of late mother has become active in the women's movement. There is nothing pathological here, but mother and father are going to have to undertake some negotiations in order to establish a new set of rules. These will affect the parents, but will also be of importance to the children. The new developments affect their lives and alter how they will deal with their parents and one another. This sort of change may create a need for readjustment which continues for a long period of time.

Most family systems have the capability to carry a certain amount of stress while new rules are being established. Even where there is a breakdown in negotiations, as long as the failures remain within the ability of the system to carry them there may be discomfort and dissatisfaction, the development of symptoms may occur, but the system will continue to operate in some fashion. This may be because the problem is of brief duration, will pass, and will permit a restoration of functioning as before. Or it may be because even a painful situation is preferable to making an important change and will be endured as long as possible. Much depends upon the resourcefulness of a given family. How does it manage day-to-day events and what knowledge, skills, personal qualities, philosophy, and the like can be drawn upon to meet the changes it encounters. For the family that is unsure of itself and feeling threatened because the neighbors do not share basic values and treat them with distance, such as might happen to a family of Puerto Rican Methodists in a neighborhood of third generation German Catholics; or the person who was the main source of family income has become disabled because of an industrial accident leaving no one in the family who is prepared to take over financial support or assume other roles; or there is no one in the family who has any great experience with giving and receiving love, so that a sense of alienation is a perennial part of the family system; these conditions create much stress and anxiety. Families undergoing such difficulties might more readily turn to rigid, stereotyped response patterns, making it difficult for them to maintain efficient functioning.

Life is easier for a family when the members are sure of where they belong and are confident of the mutual support and love of other family members. Such family members can retain flexibility in meeting new problems and resolving differences. The buffets, the pressures, the dissonances are daily affairs which may be handled with greater or less skill. There is nothing unusual about any of these situations. They are the stuff of life. The examples given do not exhaust the possibilities. Knock at any door and a family will be found trying to come to grips with life and relationships. It is misleading and unfruitful to label as pathology that which is life itself. The point cannot be emphasized enough. The challenge of life is the resolution of differences and the solving of difficult problems. Dislocations and dysfunctions occur frequently and demand responses. This is not pathology, but reality.

The fact that many situations are dealt with routinely and are given no special notice enables one to feel that all has gone well. That is not the same thing as saying there have been no problems, only that the problems have not created undue stress. It is necessary to note the fact that under the surface calm there has been a great deal happening which required actions and evoked emotional responses. Furthermore, the family members will always be making minute changes in their functioning as adjustments to the shifts made by each of the others. These adjustments account for the sense of continuity and stability within the family. In fact, the kinds of adjustive behaviors tend to be of a sort which will maintain the status quo or return the family to the status quo.

The Family Responding to Change

As has been stated, changes are a daily event. The need for responding to changes may be handled routinely so that what occurs may pass unnoticed. This may be because matters are under control and therefore nonthreatening; or because stability depends upon not noticing that there is a problem. Without a recognizable problem there is no need to do anything, of course. But persistence in denying problems does not take care of matters, and problems untended become compounded. Sometimes denial is a matter of colluding with parents. The need to be in agreement may have many aspects, but may be so strong as to prevent anyone in the family from "making waves" by acknowledging that there is something which needs to be dealt with. For example, a common family myth is that the family is self-sufficient and can manage everything for itself (Ferreira, 1963). If the basic family agreement has to do with self-sufficiency, there is a strong likelihood that problems will be denied as long as it is possible to do so. The family's sense of worth, competence, and honor are all apt to be at stake making protection of its myths of greatest importance.

But responses are not always low-key, nor are problems always denied. Sometimes the response to a problem is dramatic. There are situations where family members are producing shared dramatic responses. There are situations also where they may be producing different dramatic responses at the same time. For example: there are families who are known for their high incidence of illness and injury. They make frequent trips to the family physician and to hospital emergency rooms. Several members may be undergoing medical care at any one time. There may be, and frequently are, mixtures of emotional and physical complaints, not only within a family, but within the individual members, themselves. But whether the incidence for the family is high in terms of number, or frequency of symptoms, the emotional and/or physical well-being of any one member will have an effect upon all. This is a matter of how family members have learned to cope with stress as well as there being extra demands made upon remaining members when one member is not functioning well.

Not all families develop emotional or physical symptoms, although that is very common. Some families are notable for breaking rules. They may break family rules about many things, but they also run afoul of the police for breaking laws. The family may be involved in everything from traffic offenses to felonies and may do so persistently over generations. Some families appear to specialize in misdemeanors, while others may embrace a broad range of offenses. There may be fathers and uncles, mothers and aunts who are or have been in prison, while at the same time, the juveniles are under supervision by a juvenile court.

Many familes, of course, combine illness with acting-out. One set of symptoms does not necessarily exclude the other.

The presence of dramatic symptoms, however, does not, by itself, signify pathology. That is to say, the forms of behavior which are observed or reported do not imply that the family is sick. Rather, they are signals that there are unsolved problems which are stirring attempts to return to older patterns. Much symptomatic behavior has a reactive quality and comes to an end when the problems that triggered it are resolved. An easy matter to overlook is that there are dramas all around us all of the time. Most of them never get to court or to the clinic. These events are explained in many different ways so that their identification as dramas is obscured. And most often, the visible or the acknowledged drama is embodied in one member of the family. That person's dramatic response gets noticed even though other members may be having special problems or may also be behaving in unacceptable ways.

It is the function of the dramatic response to call attention to the fact that there is a problem. By being noticeable, forces are set in motion to correct the problems. But in being dramatic, the actor diverts attention to himself and brings the focus of attention upon himself, so that the area of concern may go unnoticed. For example, an angry, defiant, runaway child may be the object of much concern and effort by many people, but in causing a great furor may make it difficult for people to discover that an alcoholic and rejecting parent is the reason for the anger and running away. Consequently, it may be said that one of the functions of behavioral symptoms is to conceal the problem and, in doing so, protect the family from unfavorable notice. There is a paradox created by these means. On the one hand the symptom signals "my family needs help," but at the same time, so much attention is drawn that it says, "only I need help." The dilemma is too often resolved by accepting the second part while ignoring the first part. The result is another paradox: help is customarily offered to the acknowledged troubled person in such a way as to make sure that nothing changes. So long as measures are taken which have no possibility of bringing about necessary change, everyone in the family will cooperate readily. Only when the likelihood for change appears do families become wary and reluctant. It is then that great skill is required to help the family to work on its own behalf. Furthermore, until key members in the family signal that they want a change to take place, the others may be very unwilling, if not unable, to try for change. The implications here, for working successfully with families, are very important.

Axioms

Juvenile delinquency always involves the family. Every action by a family member will evoke corresponding actions by the other members of the family. This happens, not only in the face-to-face encounters between them, but also in response to what each does in the community, because such activity affects the family's standing. Accordingly, there is no way that the family of a delinquent juvenile can be uninvolved regardless of police, or other community involvement. Furthermore, despite possible expressions of indifference, family members have feelings and concerns about what the others may do. Therefore, whatever appearances may seem to be, family involvement of some sort must be assumed.

Acts of a delinquent nature not only involve the family, they make a contribution to the functioning of the family system. This second axiom enables one to focus upon how a given family is operating. For example, when parents are unable to resolve a difficulty in their relationship, there is an imbalance that results which affects the rest of the family system. Likewise, when the relationship between parent and child has become a peer relationship, or is a reversal of the roles each must have, that also creates imbalances. The failure to deal with unresolved problems in relationship, effectively and honestly, will create a blockage beyond which the family will not be successful in growing. Relationships will be limited in important ways whenever problems are not being worked on but are avoided, or an attempt is made to gain a unilaterally satisfying arrangement. Symptom development may be expected such as delinquent behavior and other signs of family stress including anxiety, psychosomatic complaints, phobias, and the like.

A block occurs when two people cannot continue to define their relationship to their mutual benefit and satisfaction. One of the consequences of an impasse of this kind is that difficult areas are bypassed and become encapsulated, but remain a source of continuing disappointment and dissatisfaction. A third party is needed to help the relationship continue. The third axiom, therefore, is that *when a juvenile becomes delinquent, there is a block in the family growth.* The occurrence of delinquent activity should direct efforts toward the discovery of what is blocking family development and how the juvenile's behavior provides the help from a third party.

The difficulty with third-party participation is, that although family members may be aware of the basic problems, it may be taboo to openly define them. This may be because the problem(s) run counter to established family myths (we have no problems, or we are a very close family); or the appearance of taking sides must be avoided; or children are expressly ruled out from commenting upon anything which has been defined as not their business; or some other reasons. As a consequence, third-party involvement may be just as inappropriate as the behavior of the two principals. Inappropriate responses, by which are meant nonproblem solving responses, will have little or no effect upon symptomatic behavior, inasmuch as the problems are not being dealt with. *Unrealistic and/or inappropriate efforts to deal with problems ensure that the problems continue.* This truism may appear to be banal, but it is not. Relationships within a family are often taken for granted, their nature considered to be obvious and self-evident. Problems, however, have been repeatedly misdefined and misunderstood because what has been thought of as obvious usually was not. Family myths, family rules, family customs may all influence how a problem is understood and defined. In turn, what course of action is available to family members will follow. The desire to maintain the status quo, or return to the status quo may be at cross purposes with what needs to take place for growth to resume.

The continuation of basic problems makes symptom formation an ongoing event. The stresses introduced into the family system by efforts to continue without resolution of the problems are very great. The effort to cope with such stresses will produce symptoms of one sort, or another. The specific symptoms may shift, but *continuation of symptomatic behavior must be considered as evidence that the situation has not been properly understood or dealt with.* It should be recognized that understanding by itself will not serve. Appropriate action is a necessary adjunct. Something must take place which helps achievement of a resolution of the problems.

These five statements may be summed up in another way: *if a youngster is delinquent, the family is having a problem it cannot resolve and the family system is under stress.* Our understanding begins with this proposition. Very often, a youngster's behavior has been taken to mean that he, or she, is giving the family a hard time. At one level, that may be true, but understanding should not end there. Accepting the premise that delinquent behavior is hard on a family may not only prevent learning and attending to what else is happening in the family, but may be a mistaken idea. Families frequently express much greater concern about other aspects of their children's lives than they do about delinquent behavior. Sometimes the involvement with the courts is too painful to bear and focusing upon school problems, or laziness, or some other concern makes things more tolerable. Sometimes subordinating delinquent behavior to other concerns expresses the hope and belief that there will be no repetition of delinquent behavior. Such concerns are understandable, but they serve to keep attention riveted upon the offender, thereby preventing a workable solution to the problem.

There are many ways in which basic problems are overlooked or avoided by defining delinquency as a one-person problem. Successful avoidance of the multiperson nature of problems will lead to continuing delinquency. For example, it will do no good to concentrate upon a juvenile's drug involvement, when the family problem is alcohol or drug abuse. It will do no good to focus upon correcting a runaway's behavior when the family method for coping with problems rests upon avoidance techniques. Neither will it do any good to work to instil respect for adults when the family style is to be disrespectful toward family members and others.

Understanding and keeping in mind the axioms, which have been stated, it is possible to gain relevant knowledge about juvenile offenses. Recognizing that the problems of the juvenile are a resultant of problems within the family system makes it possible to attend to basic issues. Actions which are developed from fundamental knowledge can be directly and logically derived from what is known and offer reasonable goals. The goals become clear and specific because the problems can be clearly and specifically defined. Instead of endless repetition of offenses with accrual of petitions from police, crowded dockets, repeated hearings and complaints from the community and/or parents; instead of repeated exhortation, threats, detention, placements and all of the other customary action; something can be done to help move the juvenile out of the justice system.

Involving the Family

What has been stated in the preceding pages provided the basis for a family approach to juvenile delinquency. Accordingly, when a juvenile is petitioned, arrangements are made for an evaluative meeting which includes the juvenile and all persons who live together at home. The reason for the meeting is given as a means for better understanding what has happened and what can be done to make sure nothing of the kind happens again.

Assembling the family, as well as other residents of the household, provides an opportunity to meet the immediately significant cast of characters; to know who they are; to begin to know what they are like, first-hand; and to begin to observe how they deal with one another. While all persons try to put their best foot forward when meeting strangers, especially those who have some official status or otherwise represent authority, the conjoint meeting with those of the dramatis personae of the family play does tend to modify the presentation and limits the extent of biased reporting. The presence of all concerned promotes greater balance and should one member present distorted and inaccurate material, someone else will offer corrective statements.

Families may anticipate that the meeting will be an extension of the court proceedings and offer argument and counterargument. It is the therapist's role to direct the meeting and to limit debate of this sort. Quarrels over "who shot John" are fruitless, so far as assisting in determining the facts. Besides, it is the court's responsibility to establish the facts. What these exchanges do provide, however, is a useful view of some of the ways in which conflicts are generated, how the various parties participate in conflict, and what the conflicts may do to help family functioning. Generally, it is neither productive nor wise to allow the family to quarrel, since such activity does nothing to alter the family's ways of coping with problems. In fact, families often use quarrels to make sure that nothing happens to bring about change, by frustrating the therapist and limiting the ability to work.

Therefore, it is necessary that the therapists be prepared to take charge. In order to do this, they have to have a repertoire of tactics for taking and maintaining control. The ability to control the progress of the meeting is necessary if the therapist is going to be able to work successfully. Each meeting has a particular goal which is to be reached, and the job of the therapist is to work toward and attain the goal. Goals differ according to the amount of time available, the number of meetings possible, and the problems of the family. All meetings are intended to be evaluative in nature and the evaluation period may consist of one to four meetings, depending upon the contractual agreement that was reached beforehand.

The evaluation is intended to provide information about the family system (how it works and who has what role). It is also intended to identify problem areas, discover unresolved problems which are blocking family growth, thereby creating dysfunctional activities, and assessing the family's situation. At the conclusion of the evaluation, the family might elect to discontinue, or make a new agreement with the therapist concerning therapy.

The approach to the family is considerate and respectful, so that care is exercised to avoid presenting the family with problems they did not know they had, or were unready to discuss. Discussion begins with a joining process—getting to know something about each person apart from the involvement in the problem. Attention is then turned to the presenting problem. The risk of commotions, quarrels, and demand for adjudication of rights and wrongs is very high here, at the point that discussion of the presenting problem is begun. The skills of the therapist in maintaining control of the session may be thoroughly challenged as the family begins to present its concerns, and any progress beyond the blaming and other attempts to arouse guilt will require much resource, lest the situation deteriorate.

This phase of evaluation, however, permits not only the opportunity to elicit the presenting problem from the point of view of each family member, but also to reformulate the problem and increase the awareness of family involvement. Frequently, during this stage the family can acknowledge that other members are having problems which are of great concern. Many times, they are very similar to those which have brought the family to attention in the first place.

Inasmuch as these families do not seek help for themselves, and a great many represent that part of the population which would not voluntarily enter into psychotherapy, a problem-solving approach is selected (Haley, 1976). This model is closest to their experience with the famiy doctor. Help is offered in the form of directives which are attuned to the identified problems. Many of these families are unable, or unwilling, to discuss any concerns which they do not understand to be directly linked to their juvenile's behavior. Despite the fact that marital problems, psychosomatic problems, or problems with other offspring are admitted, these may later be denied or ruled out as irrelevant for consideration. When other aspects contributing to family dysfunction have been identified, but the family cannot acknowledge them or deal with them, tasks may be assigned which focus upon the identified problem person, but require involvement of other family members in activities which may realign the system, or lacking that result, may bring key problem areas into the open. This usually comes about because certain difficulties between principals have been found to have prevented successful completion of the task. Exploration of the reasons the task is not carried out, or does not achieve the expected result, help to highlight those problems which are making the system dysfunctional and measures may, then, be designed to correct them.

A problem-solving approach is easily understood by clients whose confidence in the process is enhanced by having clearly defined goals with directives for activity which are related to those goals. The tasks which are assigned may not always be fully understood by the clients, but the procedures, themselves, are always clear and capable of fulfill-ment. That is, the clients may have to take on faith that what is being asked of them will help get the job done, but they can do what they are asked.

The problem-solving approach makes possible the definition of explicit, mutually agreed upon goals for the treatment. This clarity is of help in selecting means for achieving the goals. In addition, there is a way of evaluating success of the treatment, as well as of knowing when to stop. In either case, it is when the specified goals have been reached.

Not only does the method enable both clients and therapist to have some idea of where they are and where they, ultimately, are going to try to go, but it provides a structure which makes it possible to chart a course from session to session. It was found that a goal could be selected for each session. The basis for selection would be the progress of the clients to date, on their way to the treatment goals. Consequently, each meeting began with a goal and by the end of the session the goal would have been reached. According to what had transpired in the session and what still remained to be accomplished, a new goal could be chosen for the next meeting.

From the beginning to completion, there is a very clear way of proceeding which assists the therapist in maintaining control and the very requirements of the process inhibit games playing. Task assignment not only provides a way of setting important processes in motion, but also refusal to accept the task quickly exposes any activities by family members to prevent change. The contract is always being tested in ways that leave no doubt about what is taking place and allow for clarification and decision making.

Bringing the family together offers yet another advantage. It affords the opportunity to effect changes immediately in the way a family operates. When there are role reversals, as is the case with children assuming adult authority, the parent can be helped to assume adult authority with the example and support of the therapist. When the children are noisy, disruptive, inconsiderate, or rude, the parent can be assigned responsibility for monitoring behavior in the meeting. How the parents receive these task assignments and how well they carry them out yield valuable information about the way in which the family works. These directives become an important source of information about what has become dysfunctional in the family.

The work with families began with the assumption that delinquency on the part of juveniles represented a problem which could be described appropriately as a three-person problem. That is, the difficulty did not reside within the juvenile, but was the result of family problems. The designation "three-person problem" was intended to indicate the minimum number of people involved. Those persons who had the most significant input, whose involvement could affect an individual's behavior more than any other, were members of the family. In the nature of things, what parents do and how they do it, has the greatest impact; but grandparents, aunts, uncles, and siblings are not excluded. Indeed, there are many circumstances where the contribution of one of these other relatives may be very great. It goes without saying, that the juvenile deliquent's activities have a strong effect upon most families.

CASE STUDY

The Arnold family came to the attention of the juvenile court through their 15-year-old daughter, Deborah. Deborah had been arrested and charged with burglary. At the time of the arrest, she was found in possession of some amphetamines and an assortment of other pills and so she was also charged with possession of illegal substances. At the time of the arrest she managed to kick an officer while shouting obscenities and so she was charged additionally with resisting arrest and assault upon an officer. Following her adjudication as delinquent, Debbie was placed on probation. Her probation officer had met with the parents who expressed great concern over what was happening to their daughter. During this meeting, Debbie had been sullen, rude, and quarrelsome with her parents. They, in turn, had sharply expressed their disapproval of her behavior in appropriate ways with little effect beyond achieving a resentful silence. The scene was a convincing picture of an incorrigible child. A referral was made for the family to see a therapist.

Although there were two younger children, Mr. and Mrs. Arnold arrived for their appointment with Debbie. Father was looking grim, mother was looking nonchalant, while Debbie was the picture of the guilty wrong-doer. As we moved down the corridor to the office, Debbie and her mother walked ahead with heads together and arms linked. They were about the same size and were giggling like two schoolgirls. Snatches of their exchange could be heard and it was clear that sport was being made of Mr. Arnold. He bore this stoically with clenched jaw and heightened color, but said nothing.

The first order of business was to get to know the principals and it was learned that father had an important executive position with a large company. He had been associated with this firm in a middle management position and was expecting a promotion. Mrs. Arnold, despite her petite size and youthful dress and manner, looked her stated age. She was employed as an X-ray technician in a medical center, where she worked from 3:00 to 11:00 P.M. Debbie, who had resumed her scapegoat attitude, was in ninth grade where she was having problems because of insolence to teachers, failure to attend class, and violation of school rules. She expressed no interest in anything else.

That the marriage was strained had already become apparent during the walk down the corridor, despite the earlier appearance of a united front. When inquiry was made about the composition of the family and the whereabouts of the missing members it was learned that there were two younger children: Scott, aged twelve, and Marjorie, aged nine, who were in school.

Since the request had been made for the entire family, the matter of their absence was pursued and mother finally stated that she and her husband had decided that the children should not have to hear many of the things about their sister that might be discussed. It was pointed out that the children must know all there was to know. The matter was set aside to begin to explore the parental view of the problem.

Both parents complained about the fact that Debbie was using drugs, was doing badly in school, stayed away from home for days at a time and was disobedient and rude. Mr. Arnold expressed his concern for his daughter's welfare and his distress over her frequent stays away from home. He was afraid for her life and said that his anxiety over her was interfering with his efficiency at work. Mrs. Arnold also expressed her concerns stating that she had sometimes sat down to talk with Debbie about her problems. She did this by sharing a marijuana cigarette and exchanging confidences during which she learned that her daughter was not only promiscuous but was giving sexual favors in exchange for a place to stay. At this point Debbie spoke up to indicate that what she had learned during their talks was that her mother was promiscuous. She did not see that they were doing anything differently. Mr. Arnold supported Debbie, saying that his wife usually went partying after work, coming home at dawn and later, high on drugs or alcohol.

A brief, bitter exchange began which was cut short with recognition of the importance of what was being said, but a need to deal with other matters first. Mother was encouraged to talk about what her distress over Debbie was doing to her and she spoke of anxiety symptoms and frequent headaches. Debbie was unwilling to say anything at this time and was given support for being silent.

Since the time was coming to an end, another appointment was made, with the advice that the children were necessary to any further work. Mother once more objected. The realities of her fears were discussed and a bargain was struck. She would bring the children and the therapist would not reveal anything they did not already know.

Everyone was present for the second meeting. Scott and Marjorie, unlike their older sister, looked like the children of successful, upper middleclass parents. They were well-groomed, well-mannered, alert and bright with fresh faces. Some exchange was made with all members of the family and a dialogue began with Scott. In a quiet, serious voice he explained that he would like to see more of his parents. He did not see mother in the morning when he got up because she was sleeping. By the time he got home from school, she was at work. He and Marjorie would clean the house, do dishes, take care of their rooms, and do their homework. With some preparation by mother and some help from his little sister, Scott would make their supper. It turned out that father came home around 6 P.M., showered, shaved, had a drink while he changed, and went off to his mistress. This was his time with the children.

When Marjorie was asked about what she would like to have

happen, she came directly to the heart of the matter. "I wish my mother and father loved each other," she said. Such understanding on the part of those who are usually considered too young to understand is the rule, rather than the exception. If it is recognized that the delinquency of Deborah is linked to the marital distress, the family involvement is very clear.

The imbalances in a particular family are not always so readily accessible and may come to light only gradually and over a long period of time, but they can be demonstrated to be present. The fact of their existence can always be assumed, in the absence of other signs.

How does delinquency contribute to family functioning? The kinds of delinquent behavior tend to conform to established family patterns, sometimes running through several generations. Running away, aggressiveness, drugs, alcohol, and lying are typically part of family styles. Should the family be fearful of having to live by rules, it will play uproar games to prevent rules being established. Delinquency will then contribute to the commotion. In the case of the Arnold family, the parents were leading parallel lives. Mother was being a promiscuous and fancy-free adolescent, while father was involved in a liaison with another woman. The parents saw little of one another, or of the children. Debbie's activity compelled them to assume some parental responsibility and to interact with one another.

The family had not only ceased to grow, it was in danger of disintegration. As a result, Debbie was doing her best to stem the collapse and reunite the family. In the course of the consultations, however, Mrs. Arnold let it be known that she liked her freedom to be adolescent and liked her home, car, and the status of an executive's wife. She saw no reason to change anything. Mr. Arnold was strongly desirous of marrying his mistress but felt bound to maintain the family "for the children." In exploring the realities of their situation, the point was reached for a decision. They could decide to end the marriage, or reestablish it. Mrs. Arnold wanted nothing to do with either proposition, but Mr. Arnold decided to end things. A month later, looking like a new man, he appeared to announce that he was seeking a divorce.

During the early months following this decison, Debbie continued some of her activities, but at a reduced rate. When the divorce was granted the children remained with their father and Debbie completed probation successfully. The block was ended. Although, in this case the family was dissolved, a successful mending of the marrige would have affected the deliquency in the same way.

Some parents define delinquency as the court's problem. All too often the judge and probation staff agree. The predictable outcome is a long involvement with the juvenile court. The McBirney family was such a family. At the time of referral there were two children at home:

John, aged 15, and Michael, aged 12. Three older children, now adult, married, and living away from home, had, in turn, been juvenile offenders. Kevin, now 28, had been involved with the court from age 14 to 18. Anne, now 25, had been involved with the court from age 15 to 18. Margaret, now 23, had been involved with the court from age 14 to 18.

At the time of referral, Kevin had lived in California with little contact with his family. The two girls lived promiscuously and were heavily involved with drugs and alcohol, frequently demanding parental help for money and shelter. The family had persistently let it be known that the court was responsible for their children. The parents resisted referral, but finally agreed because they were afraid that their son, Michael, would follow the others into trouble.

In spite of the long, strong resistance, the family quickly got to work and was able to link their marital struggle for control to the children's difficulties. When Mrs. McBirney stopped undermining her husband, he stopped blustering. Both were able to work out an agreed policy toward the children. The next time the daughters imposed upon them, they were advised that they could move in only so long as they behaved responsibly. In turn, each daughter tested their determination and found the parents meant what they said. The daughters left. John made the same discovery and his activities tapered off. Mr. and Mrs. McBirney began a warmer, more supportive relationship together. One result was that Kevin announced he would spend Christmas with them. It was the first time in six years that he had been willing to do this. At a follow-up meeting two years later, the family was optimistic about what was happening with their daughters. They reported that the girls seemed to be functioning more responsibly on their own and were treating the parents respectfully and with consideration.

CONCLUSION

Most approaches to juvenile delinquency assume that the problem lies with the juvenile. This assumption underlies our laws, customary probation processes, and most psychotherapies, especially those based on insight. The assumption that problems such as juvenile delinquency belong to the family; that it is they who support the problem(s) and/or contribute to it as a consequence of pursuing other aims; that all family members share in the burdens created by delinquent behavior; and that it is they who must work on changing matters; shift the locus of the problem to a level which can take account of central issues, rather than peripheral symptoms. It then becomes possible to induce changes in the system, of which delinquency is a part.

REFERENCES

Ferreira, A. J. Family myth and homeostasis. *Archives of General Psychiatry,* 1963, *9.* 457–463.

Haley, J. *Problem solving therapy.* San Francisco: Jossey-Bass, 1976.

Jackson, D. D. The question of family homeostasis. *Psychiatric Quarterly Supplements,* 1957, *31.*

Matza, D. *Delinquency and drift.* New York: Wiley, 1964.

Shibutani, T. *Society and personality.* Englewood Cliffs, N.J.: Prentice-Hall, 1961.

Part IV

INTERVENTION WITH OTHER SYSTEMS

Chapter 10

CRISIS INTERVENTION WITH OFFENDERS AND EXOFFENDERS

Joanne W. Sterling, Ph.D.

Penal institutions tend quite often to victimize inmates, a process which may prevent a successful return to family and community. Increased medical problems, sexual harassment, depression, and suicide are not uncommon in many United States prisons. In this chapter, Joanne Sterling outlines the issues facing a university affiliated Mental Health/Mental Retardation Center in New Mexico in its effort to collaborate with the criminal justice system, offering important crisis-intervention programs. This collaboration resulted in a number of innovative services: a prerelease program, a sex offender program, a psychiatric clinic in jail, a court clinic, and a crisis rape center. Some case vignettes demonstrate the need for improved communication between agencies, streamlining and coordinating these interagency efforts.

THE CONTEXT

The Bernalillo County Mental Health/Mental Retardation Center (BCMH/MRC) is a comprehensive community mental health center initiated approximately 12 years ago by means of staffing and operational grants from the National Institute of Mental Health (NIMH). It has an interdisciplinary staff of close to 400 persons and a current budget of just over $8 million. It is operated by means of a joint powers agreement between the County of Bernalillo and the University of New Mexico. The county provided the original physical facility; the university, through the department of psychiatry, school of medicine, hires the staff and administers the program. Services are provided primarily to the Albuquerque/Bernalillo County area which encompasses a multicultural population of approximately 410,000 (about one-third of the total state population). In addition, the center, largely because of its university affiliation, also has become the major training and educational site for mental health-related studies in New Mexico. Over 200 students, at both graduate and undergraduate levels, obtain field work or practicum experience at BCMH/MRC annually. Students are from the departments of psychiatry, nursing, psychology, counseling, special education, and others.

Services developed over the past decade include a 44-bed inpatient unit for psychiatric patients; a 20-bed inpatient unit for alcoholics; drug abuse treatment programs; outpatient services for children; four outpatient satellite centers in various geographical and cultural neighborhoods of the city; a telephone and walk-in crisis unit which is open 24 hours a day, seven days a week; a rape crisis unit; and a variety of ancillary services. The Center provides direct services to over 10,500 people—both children and adults—annually. Indirect community education services, mainly in the area of primary prevention, are provided by the consultation and education section to several thousand other citizens and personnel of other agencies. In essence, the BCMH/MRC has become a primary focal point for mental health services and education within New Mexico.

When the Center opened in 1968, there were numerous exoffenders and their family members involved in receiving services in most of the Center's units. Initially, however, no special services were offered this high-risk population and, with time, it was noted that the dropout rate was quite high. As a result, one of the Center's staff, an exoffender himself, began a discussion group with a small number of other exoffenders. Unknowingly, a developmental process had begun which would lead to the planning and implementation of an entire forensic system during the next decade. As Fields (1977, p. 3) noted:

> In five years the Bernalillo Center has been able to help create prerelease programs for prisoners, alternative sentencing programs, therapy programs for sex offenders, a psychiatric clinic in a jail for people awaiting trial, transfer to prison, or serving short sentences for minor offenses, and a court clinic which provides

judges with psychiatric evaluations pertaining to sentencing and a person's competency to stand trial. The Center also administers a rape crisis center.

DESEO (Rehabilitation for Exoffenders)

In any event, the small discussion group, which began in 1971, triggered a series of program developments that culminated in the formalization almost ten years later of a forensic division within the Center. The discussion group spent almost a year designing a system of services which, it was felt, would meet the most basic needs of most offenders during the critical postrelease period. Essentially, an alternative model of community services for exoffenders and their families was developed. The goals of any service system, it was felt, should include the following (Sterling and Harty, 1972, p. 32):

1. to initiate a social orientation program for convicted offenders at point of entry into, rather than exit from, the correctional institution setting;
2. to provide an environment in which the convicted offender can develop self-help skills in learning to cope with the problems of everyday living;
3. to aid in the prevention of delinquency among the children of these convicted offenders, an extremely high risk group, leading to involvement with other youth of the community;
4. to increase community awareness and understanding of the problems and constructive potential of convicted offenders;
5. to assist in maintaining stability within the families of these individuals;
6. to build a base of understanding and skills within the exoffender population which will allow them to assume an increasing amount of responsibility and leadership in working within "the system" to expand and develop this basic program according to the priorities they learn to recognize and value; and ultimately
7. to explore and develop mechanisms whereby the community and the offenders might assume responsibility for the operation and financing of this program.

Consistent with the above goals, the offenders further agreed that such a program would include prerelease institutional involvement, a self-help group for wives, immediate contact with the offender upon his or her return to the community, a transitional living facility, vocational counseling and job development, a revolving loan fund, therapeutic recreation, programs for offenders' children, an intensive public education effort, and community involvement by means of volunteers and a community advisory board. Basically, this was a crisis prevention and intervention program for exoffenders. In 1972 these goals and programmatic elements were articulated in grant form and presented to the Law Enforcement Assistance Administration (LEAA) for consideration. The resultant demonstration project was funded that same year and was known as DESEO (Spanish for "I desire").

PASO (Positive Approach to Sex Offenders)

Shortly after the original DESEO grant was received, a local district court judge contacted the Center to inquire about psychiatric and psychological services for convicted sex offenders. He described problems in evaluating and determining appropriate disposition plans for such offenders, noting that they tended to be victimized when sentenced to a term in the state penitentiary. As a result, a mail survey was taken of all local district court judges. They were unanimous in feeling that sex offenders required treatment rather than a jail or penitentiary term but also felt that the community had no alternatives to offer.

Subsequently, another LEAA grant was obtained to initiate the PASO (Positive Approach to Sex Offenders) program. This program was housed in the same downtown storefront location as DESEO. PASO had a more clinical approach to treatment but its clients often participated in the various supportive services offered by DESEO.

PASO provided individual, group crisis, and family counseling to sex offenders who were referred by the courts or probation officers as part of a diversionary plan as well as aftercare services to such offenders who were released from prison or the penitentiary on parole. As Groth (1979, p. 221) has noted:

> Whatever the primary treatment plan, there also needs to be followup and aftercare services. None of the modes of therapeutic intervention currently available have proved to be cures for sexual assaultiveness. Although each may offer some help to the offender in controlling such urges, his potential for committing sexual assaults must be regarded as a chronic one, something that will need to be addressed for an extended period of time. Since a relapse will jeopardize the safety of another individual, persistent contact and supervision are required to continually assess his adjustment. Backup services need to be readily available in case of an emergency or a setback.

Consolidation

As will be recalled, one of the original goals of the DESEO program was to ultimately spin-off to administrative control by the community rather than by the mental health center. The program staff as well as the exoffenders felt that one stigma was sufficient—they did not wish to be labeled also as mental patients. Therefore, with the assistance of the advisory committee, a nonprofit corporation was established in 1975 and a community-based board of directors was set up to administer it. Known as Alternatives, Inc., the program continues to provide similar services to offenders and their families and is supported primarily with city and federal funds.

JAIL PSYCHIATRIC UNIT

Experience with the DESEO and PASO programs convinced the BCMH/MRC staff of the need for crisis intervention and treatment services within the city-county jail facility itself. As the Center gained experience in working with offenders and relating to personnel within the criminal justice system, it also slowly gained some credibility as a potential resource which might be utilized in dealing with inmates of the city-county detention center. Services were developed consistent with the principles articulated by the American Public Health Association (1976) for correctional institutions. Essentially, those principles are intended to ensure that neither the physical nor the mental health of incarcerated individuals is compromised or lost by virtue of their confinement. They also take note of the fact that incarceration may, in itself, create or intensify the need for mental health services.

Originally, inmates of the jail who were believed to be psychiatrically disturbed were transported under armed guard across town to the crisis unit at the mental health center. In addition to the potential for escape, this crisis proved to be costly since it involved, often for several hours, two guards and a vehicle. Additionally, Center staff often were frustrated in attempts to evaluate inmates without accurate behavioral data concerning the reason for the referral.

Initially, the detention center requested assistance from the mental health center with one of its most important and sensitive mental health crisis—suicides in the jail setting. The case of Danny Garcia illustrates the type of fragmented correctional and mental health systems which have and still do exist but which combine to exacerbate, rather than ameliorate, client problems.

Danny Garcia first came to the attention of the juvenile justice system at the age of ten years. He was described at that time as being incorrigible. Between then and the time his mother died when he was

13, Danny had been taken into custody five more times for a variety of offenses ranging from shoplifting to aggravated assault. After his mother's death and between the ages of 15 and 18, he was arrested for juvenile offenses on at least ten more occasions. During that period he also spent almost a year in the state facility for delinquent boys. After the age of 18, he was arrested as an adult an additional 12 times and spent a total of more than 450 days in jail within a three-year period. At the age of 21, he committed suicide in jail after being arrested and incarcerated for not being able to pay for a meal in a restaurant.

Between the age of 14 and his death, Danny had seven admissions to the Bernalillo County Mental Health/Mental Retardation Center. Upon each admission he was diagnosed as being a chronic schizophrenic, undifferentiated type. In addition, he twice underwent psychodiagnostic evaluations, one as a juvenile and once as an adult, upon the order of the District Court. Interestingly, the first of those evaluations indicated that the possibility of a suicide attempt could not be ruled out should the young man's "defenses weaken." As might be anticipated, this information was not readily available to the jail personnel who were responsible for his care and custody when he did, in fact, take his own life.

The most striking aspect of this case was the lack of any effective interaction and cooperation among the various correctional, educational, social, and health agencies with whom this individual had come into contact. Despite obvious need and relative ease of opportunities, communication was too late, if it occurred at all, cooperation was minimal, and at high stress points in the client's life, such as his mother's death, no assistance was made available from any of the agencies or institutions which had previously been involved.

In addition to the above, although there is a rather voluminous amount of literature on suicide in general, little research has been done on suicide as it relates to incarcerated individuals (Gaston, 1979). Therefore, most jail personnel are neither trained nor equipped to deal with this crisis. As a result of all the issues mentioned, the local jail administration requested early in the 1970s that DESEO and PASO staff spend a few hours weekly in the Detention Center interviewing inmates thought to be suicide risks and training the correctional officers to recognize potentially suicidal inmates. Although working relationships between the mental health and corrections personnel initially were tenuous and guarded, with time and enforced proximity each began to develop respect for the resources and skills of the other. As mutual trust developed, the jail staff began to make requests for increased mental health services to inmates other than those who were considered suicidal.

As a result, the city-county corrections department applied for, and was awarded, an LEAA grant in 1975 for the purpose of establishing a jail psychiatric unit which was located within the jail itself. The Corrections Department then subcontracted with the mental health center to staff and operate the program.

While the jail psychiatric unit staff is small (it consists of one part-time psychiatrist, one counselor, and one psychologist), it sees approximately one hundred inmates each month. Because jail terms are generally short and highly variable, and because most individuals believe incarceration itself to be a crisis, prolonged psychotherapy is seldom possible or indicated. Crisis intervention or brief therapy which assists the inmate in coping with his or her reality appears to be most practical. According to Greenstone and Leviton (1979, p. 2),

> Crisis intervention is the immediate attempt to deal with immediate problems. The major emphasis is in reestablishing pre-crisis functioning and assisting the individual to achieve higher levels of functioning as appropriate.

In addition, cooperation with other elements of the mental health center or other appropriate community agencies to provide follow-up and longer-term intervention has proved to be a most practicable approach in this context (Burgess and Lazare, 1976). Community understanding and support for this service was evidenced by the fact that a Bernalillo County grand jury report (1979) suggested expansion of services by the jail psychiatric unit to be of primary concern. Such plans are currently underway.

COURT CLINIC

Concurrent with some programmatic developments mentioned earlier in this chapter, discussions with a court administrator for the local district court led to the conclusion that development of a court clinic might be a reasonable next step. At that time, 1973, judges of the district court were concerned about dilatory tactics by some attorneys with reference to competency and sanity issues on behalf of defendents. As a result of these concerns, the district court indicated an interest in subcontracting with the BCMH/MRC for the staffing and operation of a clinic which would aid them in evaluating and arriving at dispositions for offenders. Consequently, LEAA provided the "seed money" to establish such resource.

The court clinic, established in 1974, was housed in a facility located in close proximity to the courts and immediately became involved in evaluating offenders and recommending dispositions to the courts. As expected, the ready availability of psychiatric evaluations reduced the number of insanity or incompetency pleas filed. The court clinic proved to be of such assistance to the courts that after the reduction of federal funds it was continued by means of an appropriation from the state of New Mexico to the district courts. While private psychiatrist evaluation costs were running about $116 per person, court clinic costs averaged approximately $46 per individual (Fields, 1977). The reduction in cost, as well as the ready availability of staff to perform evaluations in a timely manner, combined to extend financial support for this program beyond the LEAA grant when it was incorporated into the district court budget. This was considered to be one measure of the community's support.

ANCILLARY PROGRAMS

Several other programs of the BCMH/MRC either impact the criminal justice system directly or have some influence upon it. For example, priests, ministers, and rabbis affiliated with the Albuquerque Police Department (APD) chaplaincy program have received training through the crisis unit of the Mental Health Center. Additionally, APD cadets participate in a block of human relations training provided by the staff of the BCMH/MRC. Interestingly, this type of contribution has been ranked highest by police officers in terms of potential contributions to be made by a mental health center to a police department (Brown, Burkhart, King, and Solomon, 1977).

The Center also has a small subcontract to do psychological evaluations of offenders involved in the municipal court system. For several years, psychological evaluations also have been done on a weekly basis at the Los Lunas Correctional Center several miles south of Albuquerque. That center is a minimum security facility which is a branch of the state penitentiary. The BCMH/MRC also administers a rape crisis center (RCC) which provides crisis intervention services to over 500 victims of sexual assault per year. The RCC also has a great deal of interface with and provides training to the police and sheriff's departments, the district attorney's office, etc.

More recently, the state has provided funding to establish a small juvenile forensic evaluation team which provides psychosocial evaluations to the courts and probation offices for both juvenile offenders and CHINS (Children in Need of Supervision). Formerly, many of these children were removed from the community and remanded to a diagnostic center for a 60-day period or were released to the community with no definitive plan for follow-up services. Essentially, then, the systems' problems which have previously been identified as being crucial to the care and treatment of adults are as, if not more so (in an early intervention sense), applicable to juveniles. The recognition, by mental health as well as correctional authorities, of mutual concern in this area is crucial. It is the opinion of the author that mental health programs which purport to serve the entire community but which have not, at the same time, engaged in necessary dialogue and development of joint programming with appropriate judicial and correctional systems, are not meeting the mandate or charge which has been assigned them by the varied and many constituencies which they serve.

Mary Curtis, a well-developed attractive 14-year-old girl with a history of alcohol, inhalant abuse, verbal and physical assaultiveness, runaway, and shoplifting was seen in the county juvenile detention home by team members of the juvenile forensic unit, a component of the Bernalillo County Mental Health/Mental Retardation Center.

Mary Curtis had had a highly chaotic upbringing with essentially little structure; she was exposed to the streets throughout her early years. She was the oldest of three children born to a mother who was reportedly drug-addicted for 12 years. Her natural father, also an addict, was killed in a drug-related incident when Mary was eight-years old. The mother was divorcing her second husband who, Mary Curtis reported, sexually abused her.

Mary Curtis' younger sisters lived with the mother and Mary verbalized concern for them but asserted emphatically that she did not want to live with any of her family again. Her mother's perception of her interest in her sisters contradicted this. The mother reported Mary Curtis to be ungovernable.

The family periodically moved from state to state, so Mary Curtis' school attendance was poor as were her opportunities to learn. She was reported to be a slow learner, had been in special education classes, was reading at only a fifth-grade level, and reportedly had poor peer relationships.

Mary Curtis was enrolled in a group home, but was placed in the local detention center following several runaways, inhalant abuse, shoplifting, and assaultive behavior toward a staff member. She continued to have a great deal of anxiety and to present numerous problems while living in detention. She was unable to establish good peer relationships in either program or to use detention in a self-constructive way.

Crisis intervention counseling was initiated at the start of the evaluative study done by the juvenile forensic unit in an effort to stimulate this young woman to participate in the study and in the projected treatment plan. She was seen several times while in the detention center by the outreach crisis worker. Initially, she was uncooperative, verbalized a "stay-out-of-my-business" attitude, was uninformed and uncomprehending about the damage that could result from her inhalant abuse and lacked motivation to change her behavior as she had little expectation that her life could or would be different.

The consistency of interest expressed by a variety of agency people supporting the team approach resulted in some shift in her recalcitrance. She became more involved in planning for her admission to a residential treatment center. This, however, was quickly followed by a generalized deterioration of behavior and some activities of a bizarre nature that led to her transfer to the Children's Psychiatric Center, a state facility also operated by the university. Contact with the crisis worker has been maintained during her three months in the inpatient psychiatric facility. The worker will be available to her upon discharge to assist her in making the transition from that environment to a group home. At this writing, Mary Curtis has begun to build peer and adult relationships, has shown some relief from her former bizarre symptoms, and is substance-abuse free. More time will be needed in working with her as to how to effectively use the anticipated group home facility. Because of this timely and coordinated crisis intervention, a young adolescent whose future appeared dismal three months ago is now beginning to have the courage to risk developing interpersonal relationships and to think about a more hopeful and personally satisfying future.

CLOSING COMMENTS

In July of 1979, a forensic division of the Bernalillo County Mental Health/Mental Retardation Center was established to facilitate the administration and coordination of all of the various programs mentioned in this chapter. This is proving to be an exceedingly complex task due to the high degree of fragmentation in the goals and philosophies of the various programs, the variety of funding sources and their differing requirements, the multitude of needs of the clients served, and the scattered physical locations of the various programs.

Despite these problems, the past decade of interface between the mental health and criminal justice systems in this community has clearly demonstrated a convergence of interests; and now, as well, a convergence of efforts. The groundwork has been laid and the 1980s are expected to be a decade of increased interface and cooperation.

ADDENDUM

As an addendum to this chapter, it should be noted that in February of 1980 the New Mexico State Penitentiary underwent one of the most serious and brutal prison riots in the history of the United States. The most recent report indicates that 33 inmate deaths resulted from the riot. The state medical examiner indicated ("Causes of 26 Inmate Deaths," Albuquerque Journal, 1980) that all 33 are being treated as homicides. The fatalities, resulting from beatings, burnings, asphyxiation, stabbings, and/or mutilations, were all reportedly a consequence of the actions of other prisoners.

As a result of the prison riot, the Governor's office, the New Mexico state legislature, as well as the state citizenry are devoting increased attention to the restructuring of both penal and alternative services to offenders. The psychological impact of the riot upon the citizens of the state has been significant. Not only the riot itself, but the extreme inmate-to-inmate brutality revealed by the media in the days and weeks following the riot, has aroused the collective conscience of the state. In effect, the incident has created a crisis for all of us both as citizens and as human beings. "Crisis," as Puryear (1979, p. 18) has noted, "is a time of openness to intervention, a time of marked decrease in the defensiveness with which people protect their security and resist change." This being so, it is hoped that a higher level of functioning in the criminal justice area will be attained as a result of these recent events.

REFERENCES

American Public Health Association. *Standards for health services in correctional institutions.* Washington, D.C.: Author, 1976.

Bernalillo County Grand Jury report. No. GJ-79-2. New Mexico, December 28, 1979.

Brown, S., Burkhart, B. R., King, G. D., and Solomon, R. Roles and expectations for mental health professionals in law enforcement agencies. *American Journal of Community Psychology*, 1977, *5*(2), 207–215.

Burgess, A. W. and Lazare, A. *Community mental health: Target populations.* Englewood Cliffs, N.J.: Prentice-Hall, 1976.

Causes of 26 inmate deaths determined; 7 unsolved. *Albuquerque Journal*, February 19, 1980, p. A-11.

Drapkin, I. The prison inmate as victim, in Viano, E. C., ed. *Victims and society.* Washington, D.C.: Visage Press, 1976.

Fields, S. Courts, cops, criminals, and concern. *Innovations*, 1977, *4*(3), 2–9.

Gaston, A. W. Prisoners, in Harkoff, L. D. and Einsidler, B., eds. *Suicide: Theory and clinical aspects.* Littleton, Mass.: PSG Publishing Co., 1979.

Gordon, J. S. Alternative human services in crisis intervention. *Victimology: An international journal*, 1977, *2*(1), 22–30.

Greenstone, J. L. and Leviton, S. C. *The crisis intervener's handbook.* Dallas: Rothschild, 1979.

Groth, A. N. *Men who rape: The psychology of the offender.* New York: Plenum Press, 1979.

McKay Commission. *The official report of the New York State Special Commission on Attica,* XVI-XIX. New York: Bantam, 1972.

Modlin, H. C., Porter, L., and Benson, R. E. Mental health centers and the criminal justice system. *Hospital and Community Psychiatry,* 1976, 27(10), 716–719.

Morris, M. ed. Instead of prisons: A handbook for abolitionists. *Prison Research Education Action Project.* Syracuse, N.Y., 1976.

Puryear, D. A. *Helping people in crisis.* San Francisco: Jossey-Bass, 1979.

Schneller, D. P. Some social and psychological effects of incarceration on the families of negro prisoners. *American Journal of Correction,* 1975, 37(1), 29–33.

Schwartz, M. C. and Weintraub, J. F. The prisoner's wife: A study in crisis. *Federal Probation,* 1974, 38(4), 20–26.

Shah, S. A. Community mental health and the criminal justice system: Some issues and problems, in Monahan, J., ed. *Community mental health and the criminal justice system.* New York: Pergamon Press, 1976.

Sterling, J. W. and Harty, R. W. An alternative model of community services for ex-offenders and their families. *Federal Probation,* 1972, 36(3), 31–34.

Chapter 11

HEALING ACADEMICALLY AND EMOTIONALLY TROUBLED STUDENTS IN SCHOOL SETTINGS

Nancy Anderson
R. Thomas Marrone, M.D.

Establishing an effective therapeutic intervention system in a public school setting is no easy task. Anderson and Marrone have succeeded in developing and implementing a "Learning and Adjustment Program." In this chapter the authors describe the operation of the program and the various supportive services provided for the students, their parents, and the teachers themselves. Through the use of various case illustrations the reader can become familiar with the important aspects of the preservice and staff development programs for teachers, the educational work with parents, the team intervention approach which includes daily therapeutic discussion groups in class, and the use of various approaches aimed at helping the teachers increase their skills in dealing with and understanding the troubled students in class as well as helping the troubled student heal and change.

ESTABLISHING THERAPEUTIC INTERVENTION PROGRAMS IN THE SCHOOLS

The Learning and Adjustment Program represents services ranging from itinerant supportive help to children in the mainstream through resource rooms, to part-time classes, to self-contained classes within the regular school buildings. They include a few programs in a very restrictive setting apart from the public schools. At the present time, we operate over 120 such components serving more than 1500 children throughout the schools of Montgomery County, Pa. There are 22 school districts with a population of over 100,000 students in Montgomery County, and these 1500 children represent the most disturbed youngsters within that population (Marrone and Anderson, 1970; Anderson and Marrone, 1977, 1978, 1979).

When the program was initiated in 1964 with only one class of children, mental health professional services were sought outside the school setting. Some of the difficulties experienced in providing supportive help to regular class teachers in working with emotionally troubled children were initially experienced by the teachers in our special education, Learning and Adjustment Program. During the 1967–1968 school year, we initiated a group therapeutic program in the classrooms. We traveled to each class on a weekly basis to lead group therapeutic sessions which were designed to train the teachers and teacher aides to conduct daily therapeutic discussion groups with these children. In addition to leading the therapy sessions, we would review with the teachers and teacher aides the psychodynamics of the children, classroom management techniques, and curricular ideas. This direct support helped the teachers with the day-to-day problems the children presented and enabled them to feel comfortable in leading their own therapeutic discussion groups on a daily basis. During the course of these discussion groups, the teachers frequently expressed surprise and amazement at some of the feeling-level problems these students were able to deal with, within the school setting. As the teacher's understanding of the psychodynamics behind the behavior of the students increased, their skills and abilities to respond appropriately and effectively improved. Furthermore, the therapists' weekly work with the students in groups in the classrooms demonstrated to the teachers, through modeling of behavior, some of the ways in which they might wish to handle similar situations later in the week. This procedure also alerted the mental health professionals to some of the problems with group interactions during the course of the classroom day. Consequently, the mental health professionals and the educators gained an appreciation of each other's competencies and learned how to work together effectively. At the same time, these programs demonstrated to the administration and to the regular class teachers that it was possible to effectively treat and educate children with severe emotional problems within their buildings. As the regular education teachers saw positive changes occurring with some of the emotionally troubled children in their programs, they began to inquire about how they might assist youngsters in their classes.

At this point, it was possible to introduce inservice programming within these buildings designed to assist the regular school staff. We had discovered the key to working with regular classroom teachers, namely, to provide direct help to them for some of their troubled children in an effective manner and they become very receptive to working together with the mental health staff around these emotionally troubled children. This form of inservice, to facilitate mainstreaming of special education students, requires careful attention to timing. The reason we consider timing to be so important is the result of our own findings over the past 15 years when we have opened over 120 classes in more than 50 public schools. We found that our initial preservice presentations, although important for information and anxiety-reducing purposes, were often met politely and somewhat apathetically, since the teachers felt that these children were really not their responsibility. The preservice is important in that the administrators of the buildings are somewhat relieved to have a formal explanation of their duties, responsibilities, and role that they will play in functioning as principals of buildings wherein special education classes are located. The real benefit of the inservice to the regular faculty of a school with special education classes occurs after some time has elapsed and exposure to the youngsters and their program has taken place. At this point, some of the youngsters may have come in contact, either positively or, unfortunately negatively, with members of the faculty and staff. Regular staff may have had altercations with the children. On a more positive note, some of the teachers may have been approached by the special educational staff on behalf of the youngsters to begin mainstreaming where the youngsters can be assured of success. Then, the anxiety of the regular faculty begins to reach a rather high level. It is important to strike at this anxiety with intensive inservice and direct help to the faculty in their dealings with these youngsters. Specific recommendations, techniques, and strategies are very well received and gratefully accepted by regular faculty and staff because it has become apparent that they are in need of the tools to deal comfortably with these special educational children. The timing of these meetings or inservices is crucial. We have found, to our chagrin, that to be unresponsive at this point, allowing the situation to deteriorate, causes a buildup of negative feelings and polarization of staff within the school concerning the mainstreaming of these children which may result in negative feelings toward special education as a whole.

We found over the course of several years, that the preservice programs which we had developed for our Learning and Adjustment teachers and teacher aides are suitable for use with regular classroom teachers and administrators as well as with parents of emotionally troubled children. Although our therapists offer the most intensive and productive inservice for our teachers and aides during their weekly visits to the classrooms to run the group therapy sessions, the preservice program which incorporates psychodynamic understanding of the children and familiarizes those participants with the language we will be using to describe certain behaviors has proved very helpful.

For example, during one inservice program with regular classroom teachers on the junior high level, a teacher described the behavior of a passive-aggressive boy who was giving her difficulties and making her extremely upset and angry with him. Larry, an emotionally troubled student with a passive-aggressive personality disorder, was mainstreamed twice a week in her art class. Larry came up to the art teacher in the hall as she was about to enter the faculty room and said, "Bill gave me detention this afternoon and I'm not going to take it." Bill Jones happened to be the assistant principal and disciplinarian in that school and the art teacher's first response was to angrily say to Larry, "You mean Mr. Jones!" Larry then stated, "I'm going to a basketball game this afternoon, so I won't show up for detention and Bill will give me two hours detention tomorrow afternoon, which is okay with me." With this statement, Larry walked away to his next class leaving the art teacher feeling tremendously angry and frustrated over what to do about Larry's apparent disrespect for authority. Other teachers in the inservice program had experienced similar angry feelings toward Larry. We had the opportunity to explain to these teachers and administrators the basis for Larry's passive-aggressive behavior and appropriate treatment.

Larry's father was a highly skilled professional engineer who frequently demanded from his son more than Larry could give. His father would not tolerate "back talk" or any oppositional behavior or "mistakes" from Larry. As a result, Larry was fearful of his father and thus unable to express his anger directly to him. Over the years, Larry had learned to express his anger in disguised forms, as he had done with the art teacher. Thus, Larry had been setting up all of the people in his environment to be angry with him. We explained to the faculty that this "gotcha game" was an unconscious way in which Larry was trying to deal with his angry feelings that he could not express more directly to people. We were able to describe the stages of treatment for students with passive-aggressive personality disorders which involve: pointing out their behavior to them; helping them to realize that the reason for this behavior is unconscious anger; assisting them to recognize the origin of their anger; showing the student how they are hurting their future chances for satisfactory interpersonal relationships and job opportunities; offering to help them deal with their anger more directly; and finally, offering individual and group support to them as they attempt to change. After reviewing these stages of treatment with the faculty, we were able to offer some suggestions for dealing with Larry's behavior at the time. We encouraged the faculty not to play Larry's "gotcha game." Instead, we suggested that they reflect, without rancor, "Larry, you really seemed to me to be very 'ticked off.' I wonder if you know any reason why?" The usual response to this statement by the child is a denial of the feeling to the effect, "I'm not mad, you're all wrong" or possibly a statement that, "Yeah, I'm mad because you wouldn't let me go to the bathroom when I asked you." It is important, at that time, for the teacher to suggest again to the student that it seems that the degree of anger is more than the situation would warrant; thus, the teacher should focus on the feelings rather than becoming embroiled in the issue, i.e., the request to go to the bathroom, etc. This procedure would help the youngster to look at himself and his own behavior. After many, many repetitions of this type of interchange, it would be possible when Larry would attempt to provoke an angry response in his teacher, for the teacher to respond with good humor and warmth, "Larry, you're trying to do it again and I'm not playing your game."

Another example of a child that was discussed in this series of inservice meetings was that of Sally. Sally was a 14-year-old young lady who had an original diagnosis of hyperkinetic reaction of childhood manifested by extreme hyperactivity, impulsivity, and a real difficulty in remaining seated in the room and maintaining herself on the schedule that the school required. Her primary difficulty was that of getting into the wrong hallway, chatting with friends, boisterously calling out to a youngster in another room, and creating a nuisance within the regular school setting. Although this behavior was irritating, it was not malicious in intent and was, therefore, not seen as a particularly serious problem by the regular faculty and administration of the school. Unfortunately, Sally's father had much higher expectations of her behavior and complained bitterly about her "not acting like a young lady." This created a great deal of tension within the family and resulted in angry outbursts between Sally and her father. One week in February they had a particularly hostile exchange. Tragically, within three days of this blowup which involved the entire family taking sides, her father died suddenly of a heart attack while on a business trip to Florida. The next day, Sally came into the school showing no external effect of the tragedy except a somewhat more subdued demeanor. It was not long after that Sally's behavior patterns seemed to be regressing. Her hyperactivity increased. She performed cartwheels in the halls of the junior high school and exhibited an incredible impulse to move around the building. There was a severe and significant shift in responsiveness of Sally to the reminders to return to class or to adhere to the school rules. Whereas before, she would usually joke, smile, and adhere to the rules, now, Sally began verbal abuse and appeared to be intentionally antagonizing the vice principal of the school whose primary job it was to provide discipline and backup support on an administrative, authoritative level. This situation soon escalated into a massive and all-out war between Sally and the administration of the building, particularly this one very competent, but necessarily authoritative vice principal. In early May of that school year, Sally physically attacked this man and then ran from the school screaming a barrage of curses and destroying a number of articles of school property as she left the building. After bringing her back into the program and working intensively with her, the mental health staff and teachers of the Learning and Adjustment Program discovered that Sally was indeed, profoundly depressed, feeling incredible guilt concerning her father's death, stating overtly that "I have killed my dad and I don't deserve to live myself." Dynamically, it appeared that Sally was attempting to challenge and test the father figure in the school, i.e., the vice principal, to see whether or not he was always strong enough to really stand her assault and secondly, since he was the designated administrator of punishment, to receive from him the punishment and chastisement that she felt she so richly deserved. When these dynamics were explained to the vice principal and teaching staff and they could understand that Sally's change in behavior was a direct expression of her profound and severe depression, it became more feasible to provide the kind of structure that she needed as well as the support that she had to have. When it became clear to Sally, as time went on, that the vice principal was indeed strong, unbending, but nevertheless fair and nonvindictive, she abandoned her efforts to provoke punishment from him and began to work intensively on her problems in the group dynamic, therapeutic process. At present, Sally is much improved and, although a hyperkinetic youngster, she is not longer vicious and self-destructive in her actions. It is hoped that the normal course of the hyperkinetic syndrome which is that of gentle and slow settling will be taking place as she goes further into her adolescence.

STAFF DEVELOPMENT ACTIVITIES

We feel that in order to conduct the complete "healing system" for children with emotional troubles within a school, staff development activities for the school faculty, administrators, and other staff are imperative. We are also aware that, in the years to come, with further refinement of diagnosis and identification, many more youngsters in the mainstream of public school will be in need to assistance in the affective area. We are convinced that these problems are on the increase in light of the ever spiraling drug involvement of the young, the unacceptable loss of human life by suicide, and the high level of antisocial activity on the part of youngsters. All these are indicative of a need for an affective understanding component to be operating on the line in the public schools. Recently, we have conducted a number of staff development activities in junior and senior high schools. Although data to substantiate our overall impression are difficult to obtain, the reports that we have had from the regular faculty, parents, and youngsters within the school seem to indicate that this improved understanding, communication, and caring have paid off in a positive effect on the healing system.

Over the years, we noted that a number of extremely good teachers, skilled in their academic areas, are woefully deficient in their understanding of the dynamics of children as they pass the rough normal phases of development. Consequently, these teachers have experienced feelings of confusion, burnout, and discouragement because of their concern that they can no longer relate effectively and positively with the pupils assigned to them. We are convinced that the educational training of teachers has left this area relatively uncovered. In an effort to correct this in our inservice programs, we have offered intensive lectures as well as group discussions relating the feelings and actions of the children to their mores, standards, and value systems, and connecting these to the particular level of the youngster's personality development. For example, the developing adolescent's need to prove his independence is rooted in his own awareness and panic that soon he will be expected to function as an independent adult and therefore must reject any evidence or symbol of his dependency upon adult authority figures including both teachers and his parents. This rejection, although infuriating and confusing to his teachers, is in fact a necessary dynamic step for the youngster to go through in order to be able to function safely and capably as an independent adult. When it has been worked through with a faculty of teachers and they no longer feel that the youngster's unwillingness to accept their direction is a direct affront to them, the youngster's relationship with the teachers improves considerably. Thus, a true understanding between the generations can occur. As a result, improved teaching can take place with greater gratification to both teachers and pupils alike.

WORK WITH PARENTS

We wondered whether the mode we had used to train our special education teachers and aides and the regular school staff would be suitable for working with parents. We decided to pilot this mode with the parents of two groups of elementary-school-aged children in our Learning and Adjustment Program.

We met with these groups of parents of our emotionally disturbed children to provide them with an understanding of the psychodynamics and treatment stages which their children were undergoing. As in the case with the regular education teachers, a number of the parents were feeling angry, frustrated, and quite helpless in dealing with the behavior of their children. One bright little eight-year-old girl was able to instigate continual fights between her parents which usually resulted in their feeling guilty about having fought in front of her and finally resulting in her "getting her own way."

Stephanie's father had arranged for his family and the family of some important business clients to go together to dinner in Philadelphia. Stephanie's father told his wife that she should get Stephanie a new coat since the only one she owned looked very worn and tattered and he wanted to impress his client. Mother and Stephanie went to a local department store and proceeded to look through the coats on display. Stephanie very cleverly hunched herself over and made all but a very expensive coat look as if they did not fit her. Her mother dragged her to several other stores where Stephanie engaged in similar behavior. Since her mother realized that she could not afford the expensive coat, she gave up in frustration and anger, feeling helpless to cope with the situation. That evening, when Stephanie's father asked to see her new coat, her mother had to admit they were unable to purchase one. This stimulated a fight between father and mother with father accusing his wife of not helping with his business and of being incompetent to, "do a simple thing like go out and buy Stephanie a new coat." Mother, in retaliation for this attack, proceeded to accuse father of not making enough money to buy Stephanie a decent coat. After the fight was over, Stephanie's mother took her to the department store the next day and purchased the expensive coat which they could ill afford. Time and time again, parents reported to us these types of manipulations not recognizing that their child was angry and handling this anger in a manipulative, passive-aggressive fashion. Furthermore, as in the case of regular classroom teachers, they needed assistance in understanding how to respond effectively.

The mother of a psychotic youngster was feeling distraught, guilty, and completely overwhelmed by the profound difference between her child and the other children in the neighborhood. Her son had to be watched at all times and she felt like a prisoner in her own home. When out of the home, he would frequently run into the street without any regard to the dangers of the traffic. The parents group, together with the mental health support staff, gave both emotional support and strategies to provide for his care including work on sequential objectives to help him maintain better contact with reality. One of these objectives was to give him compulsive defenses in order to help him to cope. Mike's mother who felt so guilty about his condition that she had not previously sought any individual help or treatment for him, was supported sufficiently by the group so that she made an appointment for Mike and their whole family to be seen by a local family therapist.

Many times the child who has been identified as the one with the emotional problem is really acting as a symbol bearer of a more deep-seated and pervasive family problem involving several siblings as well as mother and father. Although this is obvious to us, we also find that most of those parents would not consider going for help either for themselves, their marriage, or for other family members. Instead, it is more comfortable to focus their concerns upon the one identified child who is in our program. Working in this context, we have approached the parents by conducting a series of nonthreatening, informational type of meetings wherein general personality and developmental dynamics are discussed with them. For example, we may present to them the characteristics of a newborn infant who demonstrates the normal "oral" dependency needs. In describing this phase we present to the parents the needs of the child at that time, his characteristics, and what they might expect of his behavior and normal development. For example, we can explain why the child who cries at 2 A.M. has no ability to wait for his feeding and no idea of the parents' need for sleep. We can explain that the child's frustration tolerance is a slow growing process and accompanies a beginning awareness of self and others. We also can point out how difficulties in passing through this stage can result in later emotional problems. Likewise, in following the child through his first several years of life, we can discuss the "anal period" which has its effect on the socialization process of youngsters as well as their acceptance of authority, expression of anger, and ability to follow basic rules set by parents and society. We can point out, for example, that this may be the period of time when a child's passive-aggressive personality traits may develop. We can suggest workable techniques whereby they can deal more effectively with their children. In this same mode we can take the children through the latency period and into adolescence describing some of the problems surrounding the adolescent rebellion, need for sexual identity clarification, and independent strivings. We have found that in taking the parents through these stages of development and pointing out to them where children can become aberrant in this normal process, that they understand more clearly the reasons behind their own children's behavior problems. As a result, discussion has been stimulated and very soon the parents become active, energetic participants who provide mutual support. To elaborate, one parent, the mother of a schizophrenic child, was constantly perplexed and dismayed by the fact that her child, who seemed to have no interest in doing what was asked of him and also no concerns for the presence of others seemed to be able to read almost anything placed in front of him and was totally preoccupied with reading books about dinosaurs. When it was explained to her that her child was desperately trying to grab hold of reality by using some type of compulsive defenses, she began to understand how his need for reading about dinosaurs was his attempt to try to gain control of his chaotic, inner world. Her increased understanding allowed her to be more sympathetic to the child's problems and in turn allowed her to encourage the family to approach this youngster and begin to break down the walls of isolation that he had built up for so many years.

Another youngster, who had been extremely repressed as a very young infant by a severe stepfather, had developed a pronounced passive-aggressive defense system to the dismay of his mother who was unable to get him to do anything "completely right." Chris would do most of the things asked of him, but always seemed to fall short of expectancy. He would forget his homework and set up innumerable situations whereby mother would be embarrassed and infuriated by Chris's inability to do quite what was expected of him. The mother sat in the parent group in tears feeling helpless and absolutely incapable of effecting any change. The support of the parent group in helping her to see that she could love her son while feeling very appropriate anger made it possible for her, for the first time, to express her feelings of anger. This anger was directed in part at Chris and his behavior but also toward her missing husband who had deserted the family. This ripple effect, which occurred as the parents understood their children's dynamics, facilitated an understanding of their own dynamics and why they were acting as they were. This particular woman had repeatedly put herself in situations where she was on the receiving end of injurious behavior, not only from others, but from her own son. The greater insight she gained through the parent groups made it possible for her to initiate changes in these relationships.

One of the interesting sidelights to running groups with parents concurrently with the weekly group therapy sessions in the classrooms with the children of these parents, was the curiosity of both groups as to what the other group was doing. We chose to not deal with this situation because of our concern to maintain confidentiality of the groups. We did wonder what would happen if we brought the parents' and children's groups together at some point in the future.

THERAPEUTIC INTERVENTION IN THE SCHOOL: A TEAM APPROACH

The healing system, which we utilized to provide for the needs of children with emotional disturbances that are too severe to be treated within the mainstream of education, is effected through a team approach. The team consists of a therapist (child psychiatrist or clinical psychologist), a social worker, a teacher, the teacher's aide, a master itinerant teacher who provides behavioral and curriculum support services, and the supervisor of special education who is responsible for the total program and functioning of the team. The team, with the exception of the supervisor, meets weekly. The supervisor joins the team every other week in order to provide a broader input in reference to program-wide considerations. The team's work begins when a student is referred to a Learning and Adjustment Program because of a serious problem or because supportive services have proved insufficient. The parents' written request for further evaluation is obtained by the local school district. The case is assigned to a program supervisor who performs the requisite paper work, collects information on the student, ascertains where vacancies exist, and dispatches a master itinerant teacher to the student's school. The master teacher then observes the child in the classroom and administers educational assessment tests. When the student and his or her parents arrive at the intermediate unit on the day of evaluation, we will already be deeply involved in the case. We will have spoken to a number of people at the pupil's school; examined his or her educational, developmental, and medical histories, and made preliminary parent contact. The psychiatrist who evaluates the pupil will be the same person who leads therapy groups on a weekly basis in the child's school district. Thus, he or she will understand the dynamics of the groups and will be able to match the student with a compatible group. Furthermore, the social worker will have a basic understanding of the student's difficulties to guide him or her in the parent interview. After the therapist conducts a psychiatric evaluation and neurological screening to determine that there is no progressive organic disorder or medically treatable problem and the social worker interviews the child's parents, everyone meets with the program supervisor to discuss the staff's recommendations. Because of the intensive prescreening involved in a referral to the intermediate unit, the youngsters we see are usually severely handicapped and would benefit from placement in the Learning and Adjustment Program. Unless the student is too out-of-control or too immature to benefit from it, we usually have him or her sit in on the final meeting of the evaluation. The presence of the child is not just a gesture, as we encourage him or her to participate in the conversation. Similarly, we believe it is important for parents to express their feelings and opinions; after the therapist explains the psychiatric evaluation, they are asked how these results correspond with their observations. The staff also discusses the operation of the Learning and Adjustment Program with the family at this time. They are told about our use of group therapy and how it will help the child deal with his or her emotional problems. We tell the parents that, if the child enters the program, they will be expected to cooperate with us in a number of ways. This includes participating in monthly parent meetings, attending periodic teacher conferences, and completing biweekly observation forms about their child's health, behavior, and home life. Our social workers cross-check the information from these parent forms with similar forms the child's teacher completes.

We encourage the parents not to make a final decision about accepting or rejecting our recommendations on the day of the evaluation. Rather we ask them to reserve judgment for a few days so they will have the opportunity to discuss the proposed placement with the concerned family members. Even if they do accept our recommendations immediately, we schedule another meeting to work out an individual educational program for the child. During this conference, the family and our staff will formulate a mutually acceptable plan to meet the child's emotional and academic needs. In selecting the most appropriate program for a child, one of the key considerations is the composition of existing groups. The team discusses the projected interactions of the group members in an attempt to avoid placing more than four aggressive or acting-out students in one classroom.

When students enter our program we direct our efforts toward three areas: their emotional problems, academic work, and family and social relationships. Our aim is to restore balance and normalcy to these aspects of the student's lives and to return the pupils to regular education when this has been accomplished. Since learning and adjustment difficulties are often related, we strive for close coordination among our teachers, aides, therapists, and social workers. To our pupils this means the therapeutic milieu of the group applies to both their academic work and social problems. The basic instructional model we use is that of diagnostic and prescriptive teaching. Because of the extensive testing and evaluation that is conducted before a student enters the program, we are able to specify and work toward well-defined educational goals. But more importantly, our knowledge of each student's dynamics permits the classroom staff to tailor their teaching to the individual personalities.

The social work staff helps with the therapeutic milieu and social interactions through individual contacts with parents and monthly group meetings. While we try to assist parents in every way possible, our social workers do not engage in long-term, intensive family therapy. Many emotionally disturbed children come from multiproblem families where there may be marital difficulties, a dead or absent parent, or other members of the family with emotional problems. This preponderance of need would test the limits of any social service staff, and it requires that boundaries be established. Outside of its normal task, our social worker program is essentially crisis-oriented. During a period of stress or extreme need, the social worker may be in contact with the family on a daily basis for several weeks. When a family is in need of more intensive counseling, the social worker will encourage them to seek outside help. If a family is receiving therapy outside the school setting, the social worker will also maintain contact with the therapist to ensure coordination between our program and the practitioner.

THERAPEUTIC DISCUSSION GROUPS

Our primary concern and efforts are directed toward an amelioration of the student's emotional problems, for we would not operate a program for emotionally disturbed children without addressing their emotional disturbances. The manner in which we do this is through weekly therapeutic discussion groups led by a mental health professional in order to train the teacher and the teacher's aide to run daily therapeutic discussion groups within their classroom. This model has been successfully in operation over the last twelve years (Marrone and Anderson, 1970; Anderson and Marrone, 1977) and is thus the mainstay of our program.

In their work as group leaders, therapists are active participants in the discussions that take place, and not just analytical monitors. We have discovered that, especially with older students, detached reflection is an unworkable posture. Students cannot relate to stone-faced therapists who never say anything beyond, "I wonder what you meant by that." Thus, when a group is discussing how they deal with feelings of anger, the therapist might volunteer that his or her remedy was to talk to a good friend. The students are permitted to determine the topics that are discussed. The therapist may initiate a self-disclosure approach when, during the early days of the school year, they break the ice with the discussion of what therapeutic groups are all about. We make it clear to the students that a group is a place where students may explore their feelings and be aware of their problems. The therapists introduce one cardinal rule of our groups, that of confidentiality. It is explicitly stated that, with the exception of when it is necessary to avoid life-threatening situations, no group member, including the mental health professionals and teachers and aides, will ever repeat anything that is said in the group to an outsider. We are quite pleased that in a program in which more than 20,000 groups have been conducted over the past 12 years students have breached confidentiality only six times.

In view of the fact that therapeutic discussion groups are a place for talking, we tell students that hitting each other or performing other acts that would be disruptive will not be allowed. It is not the mental health professional's job, however, to maintain order in the group. Rather, it is a function performed by teachers and aides. Teachers and aides are more familiar with their student's behavior, and by allowing them to maintain their classroom leadership, the group itself maintains stability. If a teacher or aide feels that a group is too wound up to continue on a certain day, it is their responsibility to express this feeling and to terminate the session. Although the situation would certainly be talked about in a postgroup discussion, it is our policy that teachers and aides are in charge during all therapeutic discussion groups. They are also the ones who handle the logistics of assembling and disbanding the group whether a mental health professional is present or not. The presence of a teacher and aide who are always in charge, gives the student in a discussion session a sense of comfort and security and fosters the handling of serious topics. We have found that this protective umbrella is the key to getting anxiety-laden students to talk about their feelings.

To encourage everyone to talk freely in group sessions, mental health professionals frequently converse with the students on topics such as sports, cars, hobbies, TV shows, or other personal interests during the early meetings of the group. It is impossible, of course, to state that after a given number of days the group will be ready to move from topical discussions into more therapeutic work. Every group is different and develops at a different rate. Some groups will be ready for serious work after only a few weeks; others may require months of preparatory sessions. Once the therapeutic work has begun, it should be noted that the group cannot sustain an intense level of feeling involvement every week. Thus, if one out of every eight sessions is assessed as being productive therapeutically, we consider these groups successful. After many weeks of training through modeling and pre- and postgroup discussions with the teachers and teacher aides, we have found many of the teachers and aides capable of being very therapeutic in their responses to the students. The training of teachers and aides, who will work with hundreds of children during their careers, to be therapeutic, has a profound effect on healing the educational system.

At this point, it might be helpful to discuss how the group assisted Trevor in dealing with his severe depression. Trevor is a 15-year-old young man whose mother had left the family when Trevor was only five years of age. His father was trying to provide a home for Trevor who was an only child. Trevor's elementary school years were marked with many incidents of acting-out behavior and difficulties with school teachers and authority figures. He had never expressed to anyone his feelings that his mother had left because, "he was bad." Trevor's father had tried to punish him but this punishment did not change the boy's behavior. At 13 years of age, in junior high school, Trevor received so many detentions and suspensions that he was promptly referred to the district psychologist who, in turn, referred him to the intermediate unit, Learning and Adjustment Program. The evaluation team immediately recognized the underlying depression which resulted in Trevor's "bad" behavior and felt that it would take several years to try to turn him around. We wanted him to recognize that his mother did not leave the family because he was a bad child and that he should not continue to engage in behavior which would bring negative attention to himself, when he desperately needed friends who could understand how badly he felt about himself.

Trevor entered the classroom group and immediately began to test the teacher and aide with behavior which was not appropriate to a school setting. Trevor always managed to get caught smoking cigarettes where this was prohibited, taking food from the cafeteria, etc. Unlike toward passive-aggressive students, the staff never felt real anger toward Trevor but rather an underlying empathy for him. The therapist explained to the teacher and aide that Trevor would have to be helped to see that because his parents "messed up their lives," there was no reason for him to "mess up his life." Initially, it would be important to "feed" Trevor in order to meet some of his primary affective needs which had remained unmet. It was also important to realize that no amount of "giving" to Trevor would be able to make up for his deprivation and loss very early in life. Thus, he would have to come to accept his past more realistically and know that he was not a "bad" child. From this point on, he could choose to engage in acceptable and appropriate behavior without having to prove continually that he was "unworthy." With this framework of understanding present, it was possible for the group to help Trevor and the other members to deal with the situation when he had stolen another student's lunch just prior to the Easter vacation break. During the therapeutic discussion group, Jody yelled at Trevor saying that she was really mad at him for having taken her lunch. Jody's boyfriend, Tim, had retaliated by tearing Trevor's shirt down the seam where there had been a small hole before. Trevor said that Tim had no right to tear his shirt and that his father would be "real mad at me when I get home because that's my only good shirt." The therapist asked other members of the group if they had any ideas about why Trevor might have taken Jody's lunch. David said that he noticed that Trevor tended to get into more trouble just before vacations and that he had had trouble before Christmas vacation, too. Jean volunteered, "Maybe Trevor's dad doesn't feed him so good when he is home and he wanted to take some extra with him." Trevor said, "My dad doesn't get home until late. I get my own meals."

Jean asked, "Who will sew your shirt for you?" The group proceeded further to explore Trevor's unmet needs and the real feelings of depression that he was experiencing. Then Trevor opened up and told the group that his father had gone to the hospital for some outpatient tests. The doctors thought he had a brain tumor. Trevor was intensely worried about what would happen to him when his father went into the hospital for surgery and more importantly, what would happen if his father should die! Other members of the group began to explore what it would mean to them if their parents were not around to take care of them. Finally, Tim said, "You can come over to my house during the vacation. We have lots of room." Several of the other students extended invitations to Trevor and the therapist praised the students for their support and understanding of him. The therapist also suggested to Trevor that when he needed help and friends, he should not steal their lunches or do things to drive his friends away from him. The social worker asked Trevor if he would want her to call his father to discuss arrangements for his stay while his father was in the hospital. Trevor indicated he would like that. The therapist gave Trevor his home and office phone numbers where he could be reached during the holidays.

During the postgroup discussion, the various team members suggested follow-up strategies for supporting Trevor through this difficult period in his life. Thus, instead of handling the surface behavior through punishment or other consequences, the group dealt with the causes of the behavior and thus effected a much more positive result.

Our goals of the group therapy are to:

1. meet the primary affective needs of children;
2. help the children verbalize rather than act out their feelings;
3. help the children understand that initially any verbalizations of feelings are acceptable;
4. help the children understand that as the groups grow in cohesiveness, they may not have patience with repetitious talking, psychotic rambling, or improbable fantasies;
5. offer the children with chronic aberrant behavior the option to change;
6. help children to understand the feelings in others that their behavior elicits;
7. help children connect their manifest affect with the true affect and its route cause;
8. assist children to monitor their expressions of feelings in accordance with reality;
9. help children change those situations they can change and

adjust or cope with those situations which they cannot change; and

10.   help the children experience support in changing or coping with situations which are causing them difficulties.

It is this group therapeutic process with a team approach working with students and parents that has proved effective in healing academically and emotionally troubled students in school settings.

Group Therapy

The group therapy mentioned above is the mainstay of our entire program and is our primary management method. The very process of encouraging verbalizations of feeling and allowing work to develop coping mechanisms to deal with these feelings makes the children less likely to have to demonstrate their problems by aberrant behavior which has been a part of their lives for so long. This process, nonetheless, takes time. During that time, necessary effective classroom management techniques must be applied while the understanding of self and others develops. For example, we are convinced that these youngsters are made extremely anxious by any lack of structure or by change in their routine. Therefore, we emphasize the need for structure within the classroom and, if at all possible, a clear schedule which does not vary. Such things as the decor and arrangement of furniture in the room are considered so as to minimize stimulation and enhance the maximal effect of the adult teacher's and aide's presence in support of the child. In the same vein, structuring is essential in the planning on the part of the teacher so that each phase of the student's day is a clear process which has a beginning and an end, operated by an individual, i.e., the teacher and aide, who are clearly in control of what is taking place. Another system that we use to our advantage is a behavioral modification technique. This is employed for two primary reasons: First, to help the youngster to begin to objectively observe his own behavior by charting and plotting his progress toward his goals. Second, to assist the teachers to be objective in their observations of youngsters and to minimize subjective comments like, "the child is sneaky" or other less helpful and derogatory statements. No small part of the behavioral modification program's effect is the obtaining of control in a class of diagnosed emotionally ill youngsters who are beset with overwhelming anxiety and are comforted by the consistent expectations of a behavioral program with clear contingencies of what is expected and what will happen if appropriate behavior is not carried out. We find that the use of behavioral modification techniques are essential at the start of new classes in the early part of the school year. In most classes, as the child progresses through the year and establishes a positive relationship with the adults, it is possible for the strict behavioral modification system to be eliminated since the children are pleased and rewarded by their own awareness that they are doing better.

We do not advocate the use of physical control; however, we make it very clear to the youngsters in the early part of the year that certain types of aggressive behavior toward themselves or others will not be tolerated and that the teacher is very capable and willing to stop and restrain any types of dangerous actions on the part of any student. This itself is comforting to the youngsters and tends to reduce the testing that might be a problem if it was not made clear to the children that control, for them, is essential to allow them to avoid hurting someone else or themselves.

The use of medications is mentioned, primarily, to make our philosophy on this issue clear. We do not feel a medication is ever indicated for the comfort of the teacher or the school where the pupil is enrolled. The medications that are prescribed are those which the FDA has approved for use in children and are indicated only in that they can relieve some of the inner pain and turmoil of the severely psychotic terrified child. Medications are used at the minimal effective dosage and discontinued when no longer necessary. In our experience, we have found no indication for the use of the "minor tranquilizers" and restrict our uses of medications to symptom pictures such as epilepsy, acute psychotic delusional states, Gilles de la Tourette syndrome, and acute hyperactivity with hyperkinesis. These measures are suggested and must be used only with the total acceptance of the family, the teachers, and the family physicians.

A final word concerning the operation of the program might be on the work of our staff to extend the measures of control which have been effective into the child's life out of his school setting. We have enlisted the parents' cooperation in managing behavioral modification techniques or other systems during the period of time the youngster is not in school, i.e., evenings, weekends, and vacations so as to provide for the youngster a total feeling of structure and consistency in all aspects of his environment.

PROGRAM OPERATION: A CASE EXAMPLE

To clarify program operation for the reader we would like to follow one boy from referral through his total programming.

Billy was referred to the intermediate unit in an emergency situation on a Friday afternoon in February as a result of the following incident: Allegedly, Billy had brought to school and distributed among a number of his fellow classmates a quantity of yellow capsules. These capsules, identified as Nembutal, were eagerly snapped up by the junior high school youngsters and ingested in quantity. The result— one child was rushed to the hospital requiring intensive care after taking six capsules and a number of other students required emergency room treatment and were discharged to their families. The incident was reported in the newspaper and on television and a public outcry ensued. The school administration was legitimately concerned about drug abuse and demanded that something be done about Billy at once.

Upon arrival at the intermediate unit office for evaluation, it was interesting to note that the school characterized Billy in rather nondescript and vague terms—isolationism, failure to be involved, and peripheral existence. Other teachers had commented upon his lack of interest in his school work and also his seeming lack of concern about his own well-being. The most insightful observations were obtained from the guidance counselor's records. She stated, "I have seen Billy, on many occasions, leaving the school in the middle of winter with no jacket, sloshing through at least three inches of slush in a pair of sneakers, his head down, and showing no awareness of obvious discomfort." It was her opinion that this seemed to be more than the usual wild abandonment of many teenage youngsters. Attempts on her part to engage Billy in a meaningful interchange were usually met with a sullen, nonparticipating shrug of the shoulders and a comment that, "nothing is wrong." On arrival at the intermediate unit office, information was obtained by the social worker who interviewed Billy's foster father. Billy's foster father devulged important details of this youngster's life. It was learned that Billy's natural father had abandoned the family when he was an infant. His natural mother was only able to keep him until about age 4. At that time, Billy was placed by Children's Aid Society in a foster home. This placement did not last and the youngster then passed through a series of three more foster homes, each terminating with a conclusion that Billy made an "unsatisfactory adjustment." His final placement occurred when the youngster was approximately age seven. He has remained in this placement to the present time. Unfortunately, his foster mother had died one year prior to the events leading up to his evaluation. An interview with Billy's foster father revealed a very interested gentleman who was obviously still suffering from his own depression and grief over the loss of his wife. At the time of the evaluation he also expressed guilt about his part in Billy's disastrous episode at school.

Billy's foster father, Mr. Brown, said that after a long period of mourning for his wife, he had finally accepted a dinner engagement with a friend. When he went to the home of the friend, he received a phone call from Billy with the statement that he had no clothes to wear for the next day. Mr. Brown told Billy he was now old enough to try to get things together. He said that he was trying to pick up his life which had been in a state of "going through the motions" since his wife's death, and that Billy should make an attempt to wash some of his school clothes on his own. Later that night when Mr. Brown returned to the home, he found that Billy had washed the clothes and father went to bed feeling good about the boy's finally taking some responsibility for himself. The next morning, Billy said he still had no clothes to wear because he had washed the clothes but did not know how to work the dryer. An argument developed between Mr. Brown and Billy concerning responsibility and "finally acting like a man." During the course of the altercation, Billy fled for a short period of time, only to return in a somewhat contrite manner. Mr. Brown drove Billy to school since he had obviously missed the school bus. According to Mr. Brown, the two "men" talked together on the way to school and there seemed to be no problems. After arriving at school, Billy divulged to his classmates that he had a bottle of pills and that he was going to take them all. Seven of his classmates swarmed upon the medication and, as it turned out, Billy was robbed of his own suicidal weapon.

A psychiatric evaluation conducted by the child psychiatrist at the intermediate unit indicated that Billy was a severely depressed young man who stated clearly that he felt that no one really cared about him and that he could not do anything right, including killing himself. Intensive interviewing at that time revealed that this youngster was suffering from profound depression with flattened affect and thought disorder strong enough to warrant a diagnosis of potential schizophrenic reaction, schizoaffective type. Although a significant and severe depressive element was present, it was felt that with intensive work on an outpatient basis, suicidal action could be prevented. The psychiatrist told Mr. Brown the seriousness of his findings and Mr. Brown agreed to become involved in supportive programming for the boy. This appeared to have an uplifting effect on Billy to the point that it was determined that he could be admitted to one of the intermediate unit's special educational programs for emotionally disturbed youngsters. In the course of the interview, it became apparent that Billy felt very frustrated and hopeless about his ability to obtain gratification from any type of significant female figure. He commented to the examiner that all the women he had ever known were unable to give him anything. He included in this statement his dead foster mother who had been the longest and most constant female figure in his life until her death one year ago. It was interesting to note that, according to Billy's foster father, the boy did not get along badly with his foster mother, although he still remained somewhat aloof from her, even after six years. However, Billy would accept her care and seemed to be quite dependent upon her for assistance in life skills beyond what might be expected for a fourteen-year-old boy.

A program placement consisting of the intermediate unit's class for children with learning and adjustment problems was offered to the boy, his foster father, and to the agency who maintained custody over the boy since he was legally in foster placement. This was accepted and preparations were made for Billy to begin work within the next few days. It was felt that speed in returning the youngster to a school situation was important since a tendency to withdraw was already in evidence from past history. In addition, constant observation by the trained teacher and staff would be better than having the youngster stay at home while his father had to go to work. Hospitalization was considered; however, it was felt that the risk would be worth taking in maintaining this youngster in the outpatient life setting rather than a more traumatic placement in a mental hospital.

The Learning and Adjustment Program social worker, armed with a checklist of affective goals completed by the evaluating psychiatrist at the time of interview, was able to explain the nature of this youngster's problems to the teacher and aide of the special education class to which Billy was going and prepare them for the types of behavior that he might exhibit. For example, although the teacher was known to be a very warm, maternal-type figure, it was also likely that Billy would not allow himself the warmth and interchange in spite of his real and great need. The teacher was advised that Billy would need constant, warm support but that he probably would not show a response in kind. In like fashion, it was noted that in the future when Billy would be assigned to regular classes, his relatedness would be much better with male teachers than with female teachers. It should be noted that one week prior to the episode precipitating his referral, Billy had been switched from a female teacher in math, where he had been causing a mild disruption by "talking too much and not paying attention," to a male teacher's class which was allegedly going O.K.

A few words might be said about the transmission of pertinent information and strategies from the psychiatric/neurologic evaluation performed at admission to the teacher who is going to work with the child in the field and in the classroom. We have found in the intermediate unit that it is often difficult for teachers to correctly extrapolate from a "standard" psychiatric report the affective goals to be used as part of the child's individualized educational plan (IEP). For this reason, we have evolved a checklist of affective goals to be completed by the psychiatrist at the time of evaluation. This checklist includes a number of items specifically stated which are appropriate goals as determined by the findings of the evaluation. It is intended to standardize, in some fashion, the vagaries of the findings of most psychiatric evaluations performed in even the best of situations.

In the case of Billy, for example, the psychiatrist chose, "will attempt to verbalize his feelings more appropriately" and "will develop more appropriate expression of feelings rather than acting with impulsive behaviors." The dynamics of this youngster's problem, i.e., his concern about never obtaining gratification of his dependency needs and resulting depression were explained by the social worker and the psychiatrist to the receiving teacher in a joint meeting when his IEP was being drawn up. In this fashion, the team members consisting of teacher, aide, psychiatrist, social worker and supervisor, were well apprised of Billy's manifest and latent problems before he entered school.

Upon entrance to the program, Billy performed as expected, remaining somewhat aloof from the rest of the children and answering the teacher's invitations to join in activities with a shrug and a tendency to put his chair back against the wall. Continued efforts were made to include him in conversations or activities. However, his privacy was respected and he was not pushed by either teacher or aide. As some time went on, Billy began to show some of his feelings by identification with some of the more boisterous and verbally aggressive youngsters. This took the form of verbal derision toward certain activities which, as long as they were not disruptive of the classroom's program, were tolerated with good humor on the teacher's part. As time went on, Billy began to draw his chair closer to the group and began to answer and participate in some of the classroom activities. In the weekly group therapy run by the child-psychiatrist, it was noted that Billy's relatedness to the male psychiatrist was quite different from his relatedness to the other members of the staff who happened to be female. It was also noted by the teacher in both pre- and postgroup discussions that Billy had established some tentative relationships with some of the male members of the faculty and staff of the school. At this point, it was felt possible to consider him for some mainstream classes. A homeroom operated by a male teacher with whom Billy had had some positive interaction was selected. In like fashion, Billy showed an interest in sports and was enrolled in the regular physical education program. His math levels were found to be high enough to allow him to function in a regular ninth-grade math class. Scheduling difficulties made it necessary for him to be placed with a female teacher who was well apprised of Billy's special needs. As Billy improved, it was felt that, although Billy continued to have difficulties in his relatedness to female figures, an attempt should be made to begin work on this problem since it was obvious that he could not maintain such aloofness. Meetings and conversations with the principal of the school and the teachers of the mainstream involved, helped them to deal with his testing of the female figures in a manner that would permit Billy to work through his difficulties in a more effective and efficient manner.

At the present time, Billy is functioning in the junior high school and is planning to go into vocational training next year. He has begun to talk about becoming "independent" and taking care of himself. In that respect, it is apparent that this youngster did suffer a profound injury as a result of maternal and early deprivation. It is also true that no amount of maternal love at this point in his life is going to remedy or fill in the gap that had been so long in forming. What we have found to be technically and dynamically possible is to work on the here-and-now, helping the youngster understand his own dynamics, and to consciously bring forth whatever efforts he may be able to muster into developing more appropriate defenses to satisfy his own needs. As Billy puts it, "to take care of myself." Billy's comment that he can take care of himself is a bittersweet occasion for everyone involved. For it means that he no longer needs our care. While the joy of returning a student to the mainstream is the predominant emotion, there is a measure of sadness on breaking the close bonds which have formed. But our goal in accepting pupils is to bring them to the point where they no longer require our assistance. We are very proud each time this happens.

Thus, we have evolved a healing system for academically and emotionally troubled students in school settings that encompasses special education, inservice to regular educators, and parent work. This holistic, ecological approach has been not only cost-effective and beneficial for the seriously emotionally troubled child, but has served as a model to foster mental health for all.

REFERENCES

Anderson, N. On the practical side, in Hyatt, R. and Rolnick, N., eds. *Teaching the Mentally Handicapped Child*. New York: Behavioral Publications, Inc., 1974.

Anderson, N. and Marrone, R. Th. Group therapy for emotionally disturbed children: A key to affective education. *American Journal of Orthopsychiatry,* 1977, *47*(1).

Anderson, N. and Marrone, R. Th. Therapeutic discussion groups in public school classes for emotionally disturbed children. *Focus on Exceptional Children,* 1979, *12*(1).

Anderson, N. and Marrone, R. Th. *The program at number twenty-three.* Book one, The program: An overview. Norristown, Pa.: Montgomery County Intermediate Unit #23, 1978.

Anderson, N. and Marrone, R. Th. *The program at number twenty-three.* Book two, The mental health professional in the school. Norristown, Pa.: Montgomery County Intermediate Unit #23, 1977.

Anderson, N. and Marrone, R. Th. *The program at number twenty-three.* Book three, The teacher in the classroom. Norristown, Pa.: Montgomery County Intermediate Unit #23, 1978.

Anderson, N. and Marrone, R. Th. *The program at number twenty-three.* Book four, The teacher and the therapeutic group. Norristown, Pa.: Montgomery County Intermediate Unit #23, 1978.

Anderson, N. and Marrone, R. Th. *The program at number twenty-three.* Book five, The child and the program. Norristown, Pa.: Montgomery County Intermediate Unit #23, 1978.

Marrone, R. Th. and Anderson, N. Innovative public school programming for emotionally disturbed children. *American Journal of Orthopsychiatry,* 1970, *49*(4).

Chapter 12

NATURAL AND HUMAN-MADE DISASTERS

Some Therapeutic and Epidemiological Implications for Crisis Intervention

Jodie Kliman, Ph.D.
Rochelle Kern, Ph.D.
Ann Kliman, M.A.

This final chapter again stresses the vital necessity of viewing the event—be it individual, family or community dysfunction—in its social context. The authors underline the importance of conceptualizing the relationship between social and psychological conditions so that the facilitations for the individual and/or the community may implement collective as well as individual mastery over an intolerable situation. Jodie Kliman posits two goals in achieving this: (*1*) expression of distress and (*2*) active mastery of distress. The underlying statement concludes that as we all are "victims," though be it "hidden," we are all responsible for acknowledging our ultimate involvement.

This chapter will provide some tentative observations and hypotheses about the differences in responses to disasters with a variety of characteristics. We will base our analysis on clinical work described in the literature of massive psychic trauma in natural and human-made disasters, on Ann Kliman's work with crisis intervention following natural disasters in Corning and Xenia, the Buffalo Creek research and our more limited and indirect involvement with the human-made disasters at Love Canal and Three Mile Island. We shall begin by reviewing what is known about general short- and long-term psychological reactions to disaster. Next, we shall examine a number of crucial variables involving the characteristics of a given disaster and the populations that disaster strikes, as well as the psychological and psychiatric epidemiological implications of those variables. Finally, we will begin to address the problem of how best to develop crisis intervention strategies that would be effective in dealing not only with the kinds of disasters which are already familiar in the literature, but with the new form of long-term, invisible disaster which has become more frequent in recent years. We do so because we believe that such disasters will become even more prevalent, increasing the need for psychological and sociological understanding of the consequences of these particular forms of disaster as well as for increased activism to prevent those disasters.

A GENERAL DESCRIPTION OF INDIVIDUAL AND COLLECTIVE RESPONSE TO DISASTER

While the focus of the present exploration is on psychological and social differences in the meaning of and response to various kinds of catastrophes, a discussion of those differences should incorporate some knowledge of common human responses to disasters of all kinds. The following description provides a review of predictable reactions to those disasters that involve confrontation with death or injury and destruction on a large scale.

In a sociological study of collective responses to disasters, Barton (1970) posits five phases of social processes involved in disaster. They are: (1) the predisaster period; (2) the period in which the disaster is detected and its threat is communicated (in those circumstances in which advance warning is possible); (3) the period of immediate, relatively unorganized reponse to the disaster itself; (4) the period of organized social response involving relief and reconstruction work; and (5) the long-run, postdisaster equilibration. While Barton's perspective is a sociological one, we can see that individual psychological responses follow the same course.

The Predisaster Period

In that period of time preceding knowledge of any imminent threat, individuals and communities tend to deny the possibility of remote threats, or to acknowledge the possibility of risk while minimizing risks to themselves and their own. Alternatively, some individuals tend to isolate the affect relating to the risk of disaster; that is, they acknowledge risk without experiencing worry. This isolation of affect is usually associated with a belief that there is nothing the individual can do in the face of a catastrophe, and with confidence that people in positions of leadership and authority will make things safe in the event of a threatened disaster. Wolfenstein (1957) suggests that neither denial nor isolation of affect is total for most people, but rather that these defenses are used intermittently in relation to remote threats, alternating with occasional awareness of risk. She also suggests that people who worry a great deal about remote threats tend to be "individuals who in their family relations experienced intense hostility together with great fear of retaliation if they expressed it" and who therefore project their fears of emotional explosiveness onto the world (Wolfenstein, 1957). Such people are likely to experience disaster as punishment for wrongdoing more intensely than other survivors. On the other hand, people who tended to deny totally any possibility of danger in the predisaster phase are more likely to be emotionally shattered by the experience of being unprotected when a disaster occurs. This is particularly so for individuals (and communities) who have had no previous experience with disaster, and who therefore maintain a sense of immunity to danger (Wolfenstein, 1957).

Detection and Communication of Disaster

The tendency to deny danger may continue into the phase in which disaster warnings are issued, particularly if the course of the disaster is uncertain and safety measures (e.g., evacuation) are inconvenient. Wolfenstein (1957) suggests that this tendency is particularly strong among Americans, who are socialized to repudiate feelings of fear, but that it also functions as a defense against overwhelming feelings of powerlessness in relation to massive danger. While Wolfenstein cautions against considering denial as pathological in and of itself, she does emphasize that it can be pathogenic if exercised in the moments immediately preceding a powerful disaster. It goes without saying that total denial can be extremely dangerous physically in the face of approaching danger.

Dynes and Quarantelli (1976) add a sociological perspective to a discussion of this stage of reaction to disaster. They report that when there is a warning of impending disaster and individuals receive warning messages, they tend to respond to the *context*, rather than the *content* of the message. By this they mean that people who are warned of danger generally take the time to check out how people they know and trust are interpreting the warning and what they are doing about it before making any final decisions (e.g., about evacuation) for themselves. The reactions of panic and irrational behavior in the face of impending danger that are so often portrayed by the popular imagination rarely materialize.

Immediate Response to Disaster

Most disaster situations, whether naturally or humanly caused, involve an initial experience of terror and a perception of abandonment by the world. Most disaster victims report believing at first that they alone had been hurt, trapped, or frightened. Regressing in response to overwhelming stress, even adults revert to magical thinking with the belief that their victimization represents punishment for unacceptable impulses or thoughts, or for some terrible misdeed. Survivors quickly recognize that they alone have not been singled out for punishment, but that they are surrounded by devastation (although some victims may go for hours or even longer trapped in such a way that there is no contact with the outside and this important recognition is therefore delayed).

The realization that one's surrounding world is no less damaged than oneself and that its capacity for providing desperately needed safety, help, and nurturance is greatly diminished at just the moment when it is most needed intensifies the victim's feeling of total abandonment (although it may also serve to decrease somewhat the sense of individual punishment (Wolfenstein, 1957; Lifton, 1967). The direct victim experiences a sense of intolerable and overwhelming abandonment and loss. Relief at surviving is contaminated with guilt over doing so at the apparent expense of those who died. The indirect victim also experiences tremendous guilt for living through the catastrophe unscathed.

For both kinds of victims, these emotions are far too overpowering in the immediate upheaval and terror of the disaster. In response to emotional and cognitive overload, victims often need to block out the impact of a too-horrible reality in order to maintain themselves for the duration of the disaster. The isolation or suppression of affect, which is also called "psychic numbing" (Krystal, 1968) or "psychic closing-off" (Lifton, 1967), allows victims (and, as we shall see, rescue workers and other "hidden victims") to go about the essential business of rescuing their fellows, caring for the injured, and the dependent, viewing or handling the dead and so forth without being overwhelmed and rendered impotent as a result of total immersion in death, pain, and destruction. This psychic numbing is functional during the crisis itself. It may be transient, or it can continue indefinitely, merging with the depression and despair that is characteristic of the "survivor syndrome" (Lifton, 1967).

Prolonged psychic closing-off is far more likely to occur in response to particularly all-encompassing human-made disasters, such as those experienced by Jews during the Holocaust and the people of Hiroshima and Nagasaki after their cities were bombed. Generally, in natural disasters, psychic numbing in its more extreme forms does not last more than the first hour or so beyond the initial impact of the disaster, and then only for a small proportion of the population. The numbing that does occur for the most part does not interfere with appropriate behavior immediately following the disaster impact. Barton (1970) reports that following a tornado in Arkansas, five percent of the men and one-third of the women were "dazed" during the first half hour and that most of them were able to function appropriately at the end of that half-hour period.

Popular belief has it that in disaster, chaos and panic prevail, along with an "every man for himself" attitude among the stricken populations. Virtually all the research on disaster responses paint a very different picture. Most victims of disaster report either helping others or being helped, and a sense of solidarity, altruism, and support within the affected community. The only situations in which this solidarity and mutual help is not the primary collective response are those in which people killed or injured greatly outnumber those in a position to be helpful, as occurred in Hiroshima, or in which escape routes are in view but blocked off, so that panic and trampling ensue, as occurs in some hotel fires.

Wolfenstein (1957) and Lifton (1967) suggest that the sense of solidarity and altruism, or "postdisaster utopia" that begins in the first hours following the actual impact of a disaster serves an important psychological function. As previously mentioned, the direct victim's initial response to the catastrophe involves the belief that he/she has been punished for some serious misdeed or wickedness. Tremendous relief accompanies the realization that one has survived, that the ultimate punishment was not carried out. This relief is guilt-provoking, however, if others have been more seriously wounded or killed, because the relief involves an emotionally unacceptable gladness that it is others, and not oneself who died. This guilt is shared by indirect victims, who tend on an unconscious level to view the disaster as a punishment which was meant for them but which they evaded. Guilt over one's desire to survive, which survivors perceive as at the expense of others, combines with the mystifying and magical quality of the disaster itself to evoke the fear that the disaster will reoccur and that next time it will be impossible to avoid the just punishment of death.

Under these circumstances, doing good for others is the ideal atonement for one's perceived selfishness and guilt and can be used to strike a safe bargain with the punitive powers that be. It is psychologically imperative to find ways to see oneself as good again, and therefore as safe from further harm. This dynamic nicely complements that of the more severely hurt or otherwise more dependent direct victims. In the initial phase of the disaster, the direct victim who is hurt or otherwise incapacitated feels an absolute sense of abandonment by the world. When subsequent help is offered, the victim is immensely grateful because help and attention prove that the world can still provide essential nurturance after all. This gratitude, in turn, helps the guilt-ridden helper to feel less selfish and bad, and therefore safer from future punishment.

Finally, Wolfenstein (1957) suggests that the damage wrought by the disaster provides people with a vicarious gratification of aggressive impulses. Once this gratification is achieved, the positive side of ambivalent relationships to members of one's own social network and to people in general is activated. As a result, disaster victims report feeling great surges of love for family, friends, acquaintances, and even strangers.

Organized Response to Disaster

As the immediacy of the initial catastrophe passes, the rescue work is completed and the extent of damage and loss experienced by the community and its members is known, a new phase of psychological and social response to disaster begins. For most individuals, psychic numbing begins to wear off and powerful emotions emerge. This process of reentering emotional life is similar to that experienced in the mourning of a death; overwhelming feelings of loss and grief are not allowed until they can be managed in gradual doses. Most disaster victims do not relinquish the defense of numbing all at once; rather, they slowly let their feelings into consciousness. Some do not lower their defenses for some time.

Disaster victims—and victims of any trauma—frequently experience considerable anxiety over the possibility that the disaster might recur. They find themselves brooding over this possibility and over what they would do to keep themselves and their loved ones safe in the event of recurrence. They repeatedly relive the original trauma in their imaginations. Although these thoughts are generally frightening and feel out of control, they serve a mastery function, gradually inuring the victim to the overpowering impact of disaster experience. Through these repetitious thoughts, the disaster victim slowly develops an ability to deal on an affective level with an experience that, up to this point, was psychologically too dangerous to process completely.

In addition to the "passive" mastery of the disaster trauma through repeated thoughts and fantasies, many disaster victims utilize the "active" mastery entailed in talking about the disaster.

As the defenses of psychic numbing and denial are exercised less powerfully, the horrors of the catastrophe take on a sense of reality for the victims. It is at this point (with the exception of massive human-made disasters such as atomic bombings or concentration camps) that symptomatology may develop. Most of the psychological or psychogenic symptoms that emerge at this point are transient in nature, but they can be longer lasting in a significant minority of victims. Barton found that following an Arkansas tornado, almost 90 percent of the adults in the impact area and 70 percent of those not directly affected reported suffering minor disturbances such as sleeplessness, lack of appetite, headaches, preoccupation with the storm, inability to concentrate, nervousness, hypersensitivity to storm cues, etc., in the first two weeks after the tornado struck. Of the direct and indirect victims reporting symptoms, only about one-sixth in either group indicated that their ability to work was interfered with as a result (Barton, 1970).

So long as psychic numbing and denial continue, disaster victims can believe on some level that the calamity that befell them is merely a prolonged and frightening dream from which they will awake. That defensive belief dissipates as days and weeks go by and the aftermath of the disaster lingers on. Loved ones whose deaths could not be assimilated do not reappear, destroyed homes remain in shambles, temporary shelters are cramped and impersonal and allow no privacy—the disaster situation defies a return to normalcy.

As this painful reality becomes inescapable, dependency needs intensify and direct victims become increasingly demanding of others. Their demands often appear unreasonable in contrast with their earlier, grateful acceptance of whatever little assistance could be offered, and indirect victims and official caregivers (who constitute the "hidden victims" of the disaster) begin to lose patience with the direct victims' complaints and neediness. Direct victims' attempts at mastery of intolerable experiences through repeated discussion of those experiences become increasingly difficult for the indirect victims, whose growing impulse is to avoid thoughts of the disaster, to hear. At the same time, the original emergency is replaced by its long-term aftereffects and indirect victims and caregivers find fewer ways to be of practical help to direct victims. Their guilt-reducing helpful activity can no longer find as many established outlets. In response to increasing demands, coupled with a decrease in an objective ability to help, indirect and hidden victims begin to pull away from direct victims and to try and restabilize their own lives just as the direct victims begin to feel most deprived and cheated.

A conflictual division is thus established between the people who have been affected directly by the catastrophe and those who are indirectly affected. Direct victims come to resent those who lived through the disaster without harm and who are beginning to return to relatively normal lives when their own lives are so completely disrupted. Indirect victims and caregivers want to help and feel guilty toward those who were directly affected, but resent the impossible demands made on them and begin to think that perhaps the direct victims are weak, malingering, or taking advantage of the situation. The postdisaster utopia commences its decline with this divisiveness.

During the earliest stages of reaction to disaster, rescue work and other help are usually provided on a relatively unorganized basis by community members, most often by members of the victims' own social networks. After the first hours and days, however, the bulk of this work is turned over to established governmental, social, and voluntary agencies. While some of these agencies may be staffed by known community residents, most represent the "outside." These agencies vary in the degree to which they are bureaucratic—a characteristic which is relatively absent in the initial, community-based rescue efforts. The nature of the services provided also changes. Concerns for immediate safety, which are acted upon personally and without delay, are replaced by concerns for federal loans and grants for rebuilding, insurance payments, long-term medical and legal entanglements, etc., all of which entail delays, red tape, and conflict between victims and representatives of outside, bureaucratic agencies.

Once the immediate emergency has subsided and long-range planning becomes central to rehabilitation work, various local and governmental agencies predictably come into conflict over "ownership" and "territorial rights" over the postdisaster process. Old rifts widen and competitions intensify as different agencies struggle to regain functions that were shared during the emergency but which previously had belonged to them or which had been objects of territorial dispute (Kliman, 1976). Another dynamic which may be at work here is that caregivers frequently displace their countertransferential frustration with victims onto other caregivers, rather than acknowledging their guilt-provoking feelings about "those poor people."

Not surprisingly, conflict emerges on a political level as well. In this fourth phase of disaster response, political structures reassert their control after a relatively anarchic time during which unofficial groups and collectivities defined much of community strategy for managing the early stages of the crisis. Brown and Goldin (1979) argue that the reconsolidation of official control stands in necessary conflict with the continued existence of the unofficial groupings as agents in postdisaster politics, and has as its goal the reestablishment of the predisaster political *status quo*.

A key struggle between official and unofficial organizations often concerns the assignment of responsibility for the disaster (or its potential avoidance), and of credit or blame for postdisaster events. These struggles generally involve individuals (e.g., elected officials) rather than structures, "because the only possible political outcome envisaged is in terms of retaining or replacing specific operators rather than in terms of revising the social order itself" (Brown and Goldin, 1979). This struggle can be conceptualized as part and parcel of the vying for control described above, because the definition and allocation of responsibility relate directly to the hierarchy of control within any social system.

On another level, the informal mutual help that characterizes the early phases of the disaster need not compromise the victims' desire to maintain some degree of autonomy despite their situation (Wolfenstein, 1957). The unilateral and impersonal quality of official help during the postdisaster reconstruction effort, on the other hand, intensifies victims' sensitivity to their unwelcome dependence upon others. It also leads victims to suspect that help they receive is "counterfeit" nurturance. Heightened awareness of an ambivalently experienced dependence, in conjunction with the generally inadequate official response to the physical, economic, and psychological neediness of victims, exacerbates the underlying conflict between victims and the structures of official (i.e., economic and political) control.

Postdisaster Equilibration

This final stage involves the slow return to predisaster status following the psychological and social upheaval of the first four phases of the disaster. For many direct and indirect victims, this new situation is close to that which preceded the disaster experience, although some relatively encapsulated psychological sequelae may be maintained (e.g., fright at the sound of a storm for a hurricane victim) for years afterward. For those who were particularly hard-hit emotionally, for instance, people who were multiply bereaved or whose preexisting psychological disturbances were compounded by the disaster, the sequelae may be more damaging and long-lived.

Social agencies that entered into competitive relationships during the earlier stages of the disaster, or whose competition was intensified during that time, tend to remain divided once a postdisaster situation is attained. The results of Ann Kliman's community intervention with a variety of social agencies in Corning suggests that the crisis situation generated by disaster has the potential to be used effectively to establish higher levels of interagency cooperation (Kliman, 1976). However, this positive development is unlikely to occur without careful and energetic consultative and facilitative work.

The domination of communication and information (largely through the local media) by official structures of control is crucial to the reestablishment of the social order of the predisaster period. This is particularly true in the event of a human-made catastrophe or natural disaster which might have been averted through human effort. The assertion of control over postdisaster information and influence over prevailing beliefs concerning the management of disaster further legitimates and empowers established authority.

Schiller (1973) describes how the media report isolated facts in such a way that they are trivialized and cannot easily be synthesized for a complete and integrated understanding of a given phenomenon. Such a presentation renders the formulation of a critical analysis of the established order difficult, especially for the victims who lack alternative resources for understanding the disaster in its full social context. This kind of manipulation of information and belief systems is likely to occur in the wake of a disaster—particularly if those in control can be justifiably criticized for their part in the disaster or its aftermath, or if the momentary egalitarianism of the "postdisaster utopia" threatens the longevity of the social order.

A concrete example of this return to the old order is seen in the following typical postdisaster scenario: The families of a well-to-do homeowner and a working-class poor apartment tenant are both displaced by a tornado and for a short period live side by side in a temporary shelter the Federal Government has set up in trailers. The wealthier family receives insurance benefits and federal low-interest loans for rebuilding and they resume their original standard of living, while the second family, who have lost all their worldly possessions, do not qualify for financial help because they are not homeowners. This family ends up in worse financial shape than ever, but their economic backslide is justified bureaucratically.

SOME PSYCHIATRIC EPIDEMIOLOGICAL VARIABLES CONCERNING THE CHARACTERISTICS OF DISASTERS AND DISASTER POPULATIONS

We move now to an examination of some of the salient characteristics of disasters and their victims. We identify eight variables in this analysis, addressing characteristics of the disasters, the populations affected, and the relation between them. We draw on materials on various communities in disaster as we are concerned with understanding the effects of different types of collectively experienced disasters on different types of populations. While our primary focus in on populations rather than individuals, it will also be important to pay attention to the effects of individual variables, such as preexisting psychopathology, on long-term psychological functioning following the disaster experience.

The first four variables to be addressed deal with characteristics of the disaster itself: (*1*) whether the disaster is natural or human in its origin; (*2*) whether, if the disaster is human-made, it is the result of (a) an intentional act of aggression; (b) an unpredictable accident; (c) a predictable accident; or (d) a chronic situation which is not recognized as dangerous until after the damage is done; (*3*) whether the disaster is time-limited or ongoing in nature, and (*4*) the extent of damage, including the ratio of directly affected to indirectly affected populations.

A fifth variable concerns the relation between the disaster and the population it strikes: (*5*) if the disaster is human in origin, whether the relationship between the victims and the agents of the disaster is such that (a) victims and agents of the disaster have no previous relationship (e.g., in an airplane crash); (b) the agents of the disaster are outsiders or enemies of the victims (e.g., in wartime bombing); or (c) the affected community is historically dependent in some way (e.g., economically) on those responsible for the calamity.

The remaining variables relate to the psychological and social characteristics of the individuals and populations affected by the disaster: (*6*) the individual's level of psychological functioning and conflict prior to the onset of the disaster; (*7*) whether the individual is a direct victim, indirect victim, or caregiver (hidden victim); and (*8*) the class and gender position of the victim.

It is, of course, necessary to omit many variables from this analysis for the sake of achieving some degree of focus and so these eight variables in no way comprise an exhaustive list. Some variables which merit exploration but cannot be addressed here include: psychological development of the individual victim, such cross-cultural factors as values concerning altruism and dependency, religious and political belief systems; the economic and political system in which the disaster and disaster management are imbedded; and prior experience with disaster and disaster preparedness on the part of individuals and communities.

Natural versus Human-Made Disasters

The first variable concerns the causation of disaster, that is, whether it is the result of natural or human forces. Lifton and Olson's (1976) study of psychological reactions to the catastrophic dam collapse in Buffalo Creek describes victims as significantly less able to master the experience of confrontation with widespread death following this flood than victims of floods which were equally devastating but naturally caused. They point out that "in many [natural] disasters survivors are able to find some comfort, or at least resignation, in the deep conviction that what happened was a matter of God's will, or of some larger power that no mortal could influence," but that such consolation was not possible among the survivors of a disaster that was caused and could have been prevented by man (Lifton and Olson, 1976).

These authors report that virtually all the Buffalo Creek survivors they interviewed experienced an inversion of their moral world, "of wrongdoings going unpunished and responsibility unacknowledged while innocent victims undergo pain and suffering," which provided obstacles to mastery and resolution of the traumatic experience and left survivors bitter and confused: "They remain locked in the death anxiety, survivor guilt, numbing and impaired relationships, bound to the disaster itself and to its destructive psychological influences" (Lifton and Olson, 1976, p. 303).

It frequently happens, with the occasional exceptions of intentional destruction, that victims of the disaster have great difficulty finding outlets and clear targets for their rage at victimization.

In addition to the depression-inducing internalization of rage, victims of human-made disasters tend to see themselves as deserving the punishment meted out to them by disaster, in the conscious or unconscious belief that no one would *allow* such a thing to happen to someone who is valuable as a human being. This loss of self-worth is likely to be particularly strong for someone who had already internalized a sense of worthlessness before the disaster, as happens in a lifetime of exploitation and of a reduction of human value to one's productive output. Lifton and Olson (1976) convincingly argue that "people who feel their humanity violated and unrecognized by others internalize that diminished sense of themselves in ways that impair the capacity for recovery or even hope." Lifton (1976) describes a Hiroshima survivor, "a downtrodden woman laborer, middle-aged and alone in life" when badly injured in the bombing, who was brought to a medical facility and left virtually unattended for a week. "As one accustomed to neglect, she stifled her rage at first and even justified her being ignored, but was soon overcome by feelings of worthlessness as virtually to reach out for death" (Lifton, 1967, p. 44).

The experience of another person's death inevitably leads to some degree of survivor guilt. The greater intensity of this guilt in response to deaths experienced on a larger scale in natural disasters is well documented (Lindemann, 1944; Wolfenstein, 1957; Kliman, 1976). This guilt and the above-described feelings of worthlessness serve to activate and compound each other in human-made disaster (Lifton, 1967; Krystal, 1968; Lifton and Olson, 1976).

There are significant differences in social and political responses to natural versus human-made disasters. Brown and Goldin's description of the reassertion of official control following the initial stages of the postdisaster period is discussed in the preceding section. Their description can be expanded by pointing out that when those in political or economic power can be held responsible in any way *for the disaster itself*, and not merely for the management of its aftereffects, their need for control over the information and ideological views disseminated to the public is greatly increased.

A chilling example of authorities' manipulative and even propagandistic control over disaster information is found in official reports to the local and national news media concerning the continuing dangers at the Three Mile Island nuclear power plant. For the 11 months after the accident, officials of the utility company and the Nuclear Regulatory Commission denied that radioactive gases were being released into the atmosphere, despite clear-cut evidence to the contrary (high geiger-counter readings kept by private citizens, a metallic taste in the mouths of many residents on the days the readings went up, etc.). When the emissions were finally acknowledged, just prior to the first anniversary of the accident, they were declared to be perfectly harmless, along with the radiation released at the time of the accident itself. This declaration stood in stark contradiction to the accumulating medical evidence of staggering increases (still denied by many official sources) in the rates of infant mortality, birth defects, and thyroid conditions among the human population and the ubiquitous deaths, stillbirths, and birth defects among livestock and outdoor pets since the accident (Cowan, 1980; Leaser, 1980; Timkoe, 1980; Franklin, 1980).

When such an obvious manipulation and covering up of the facts comes to light, it has important repercussions on the ability of official reports and reassurances to elicit trust among the public. When a mother learns that she has been deceived about the contamination of air and water supply, why should she believe official reassurances that her child's high body scan (for radiation) is nothing to worry about? Under such circumstances, many people who never previously examined official ideologies critically may begin to do so.

Causes of Human-Made Disaster

Human-made disasters can be categorized by causality, a variable which is significant in terms of victims' social and psychological relationships to the catastrophe.

a. The first and most devastating category of human-caused disaster involves those destructions of life and property that result from acts of aggression, as happens in war. The particular horror of massive exposure to death, loss, and damage is greatly compounded by the awareness that this devastation was intended by other human beings. The tendency to view the abandonment and loss entailed in disaster as a punishment and to accept a view of oneself as worthless is exaggerated when there is, in fact, an agent of punishment to be found. Lifton (1967), in his study of Hiroshima survivors, and Niederland (1968) and Krystal (1968) in their clinical work with concentration camp survivors years after World War II found a consistent profile including nagging feelings of survivor guilt, worthlessness, depression, and suspiciousness of others. While there is considerable epidemiological evidence that long-term psychological functioning after disaster correlates highly with the degree of previous emotional conflict or disturbance, this does not appear to be the case for the psychological sequelae of massive war trauma. Rather, this experience is so overwhelming that previously high levels of functioning do not seem to be adequate insurance against the effects of such massive trauma.

   b. The second category of human-made disaster encompasses those resulting from unpredictable accidents, such as airplane crashes involving human error, rather than structural failure. While we have little information on this kind of disaster, we hypothesize that it has fewer emotional consequences, all other things being equal, than other forms of disaster resulting from human action.

   c. The third category of human-made disaster includes those accidents which are predictable, but are nevertheless risked (usually for economic reasons). Examples of this type of disaster are found in the nuclear accident at Three Mile Island, where the buildup of the "hydrogen bubble" which started the accident was a known risk; the collapse of a faulty dam at Buffalo Creek; the 1978 mid-air collision over San Diego Airport, where traffic controllers, among others, had complained for years about the risks involved in the airport tracking system and; the DC-10 crashes that occurred after the discovery of a structural defect in those planes. Lifton and Olson poignantly describe the emotional implications of the understanding that one's life has knowingly been risked by others for the sake of profit. Whereas most of the victims of naturally occurring floods ultimately are able to bury their dead, nurse their wounded, rebuild their homes, and come to some degree of psychological resolution of their losses, the ability to reenter life and complete the process of mourning is severely impaired under the circumstances of a human-caused disaster. A kind of "death-in-life" prevails among Buffalo Creek survivors, a depressed and despairing outlook resembling that of wartime victims.

   d. The last type of human-made disaster to be discussed involves a chronic situation in which the physical environment is dangerously altered over a relatively long period of time, with the recognition of danger coming only after the damage is done. One example is seen in Love Canal, Niagara Falls, a dumping ground for chemical wastes for decades which subsequently was ground-filled and converted into acreage for homes. Years after the homes had been built and inhabited, several of the chemical wastes were found to be carcinogenic or otherwise harmful and to be leaching into the people's homes.

In this situation, there is no earthquake, no approaching wall of water, no explosion on which to pin immediate fear. Rather, there is the sudden realization that one has been in danger for a long time, possibly made sick as a result, and certainly at high risk for future illness. It is more difficult in such a situation to find a clear target for anger than in other forms of human-made disaster, because the risk of disaster was taken in ignorance. Under these circumstances, any rage that is felt is likely to be experienced as inappropriate or irrational, except when directed at present behavior, such as the attempt by the government and chemical companies at Love Canal to avoid the costs of moving endangered residents and paying their medical expenses. This kind of situation quickly settles into a despairing and paralyzing chronicity in much the same way as an urban ghetto (which is also a product of the economic and political system and hazardous to the health of its populations).

Our frustrating and saddening experience in consulting with the United Way agencies at Love Canal was that the murkiness and pessimism of the situation resulted in divisions among victims: between those whose homes were so situated that the government was forced to take responsibility for moving them and those equally endangered residents who, by virtue of arbitrary geographic demarcations, were not eligible for relocation, and between homeowners and apartment dwellers. Effective community organization was nearly impossible in an atmosphere of hopelessness and misplaced conflict. Conflict was manifested between spouses, between neighbors and between helping agencies (Maloney, 1980). No one seemed quite sure how to take on more appropriate but formidable opponents like Hooker Chemical a subsidiary of an enormous multinational corporation, Occidental Petroleum, responsible for much of the chemical dumping, and the United States government.

Time-Limited versus Chronic Disasters

The period of time over which the effects of a disaster last is crucial to the ultimate resolution of the disaster—and, in many cases, to the health and safety of the survivors. Most natural disasters are brief in duration, lasting minutes or hours and leaving predictable and finite aftereffects. While this is true for certain human-made disasters, the aftereffects of some continue for years. The effects of radiation at the sites of atomic bombings or tests, and accidents like the one at Three Mile Island can go on for generations, since many radioactive isotopes have long half-lives. The contamination of the environment by toxic or carcinogenic wastes similarly lasts even beyond the lifetime of the original victims.

An important psychological difference between "acute" and "chronic" disasters is that the latter involve the sense of ongoing danger to oneself and one's loved ones. In Hiroshima, where radiation-related diseases such as leukemia and the vague, ubiquitous and all-inclusive "A-bomb disease" may not have been manifested for years, almost every minor ailment becomes cause for concern over the effects of the invisible contamination. "Survivors felt themselves involved in an endless chain of potentially lethal impairment which, if it does not manifest itself in one year—or in one generation—may well make itself felt in the next" (Lifton, 1967, p. 130). The physical effects of the radiation were real, terrifyingly widespread, and seemingly limitless. This mysterious and on-going medical risk had a powerful influence on the psychologies of Hiroshima survivors. In addition to the physical sequelae of the bomb's explosion, Hiroshima physicians reported an endemic "A-bomb neurosis," involving a life-long preoccupation with radiation-related disease. While not enough time has elapsed since the nuclear accident to determine long-term effects (e.g., rises in cancer rates), physicians in the vicinity of Three Mile Island have been reporting major increases in physical symptoms, such as gastrointestinal distress, headaches, fatigue, insomnia, and rashes, some of which could be directly related to radiation exposure, but which are also likely to be stress-related and psychogenic. Under circumstances which are simultaneously emotionally stressful and physically dangerous, attempts at ascertaining etiology are confounded. Short-term psychological effects are clear, however; the Pennsylvania Health Department recently reported that for people living within 15 miles of the reactor, there was a 113% increase in use of sleeping pills and an 88% increase for tranquilizers, while 14% increased their alcohol consumption and 32% smoked more cigarettes than before the accident (Franklin, 1980; Leaser, 1980).

Another crucial issue relating to this variable involves the psychological and medical implications of the choice (if a true choice is possible) between leaving or remaining in the affected area. Most of the endangered residents of Love Canal have, after a long struggle with government officials, left their homes, but many question their safety in a region which is rife with chemical dumping grounds. In contrast, few have left the immediate vicinity of Three Mile Island (radioactive gases in the atmosphere travel farther than underground chemicals), despite the growing awareness of the dangers in staying. Much of this decision is economic—it is not easy to give up a home that can no longer be sold and which has a 6% mortgage to buy a house somewhere far away, with a 20% mortgage if a mortgage is even possible. It is also hard to leave one's roots behind. Children and adults have social networks and memories which provide strong emotional ties to their homes.

Most of the people who stay exercise a continuous or intermittent denial ("We are safe because we live five miles from the plant and we mostly stay indoors") or an isolation of affect ("We've already been exposed and there is nothing we can do anyway") in order to tolerate the reality of staying. Some people choose to stay in order to fight it out, like David against Goliath, accepting a measure of danger in order to "catch the nuclear villains" at their deadly game (Timkoe, 1980). The emotional price, and perhaps the medical one, is high.

Extent of Damage

Simply put, the greater the number of people directly suffering loss or injury in a disaster in proportion to those not directly affected, the less direct victims will be able to receive immediate and adequate help or, if they are not badly injured, to provide help. Thus, the higher the proportion of direct victims, the greater the devastation and sense of abandonment, the more massive the trauma experienced by victims and the worse the long-term effects may be. Not coincidentally, the more pervasive and devastating catastrophes are likely to be human in origin.

The Relationship Between Victims and Agents of Human-Made Disaster

There are three kinds of relationships between disaster victims and those responsible for the disaster.

a. The first, and least psychologically conflictual relationship is one in which the disaster victims and the agents of the disaster have no prior connection with each other. An example of this situation is seen in commercial airline crashes, in which there is no significant relationship between the airline or the plane manufacturer and the crash victims. Anger can be expressed and there is less feeling that one's life is held unimportant. Although only few data are available to back up this hypothesis, we suspect that the emotional sequelae of this kind of disaster should be considerably less severe than for other human-made disasters and may more closely follow the psychological sequelae of natural disaster.

b. A second possible relationship is one in which the agents of destruction stand outside the stricken community, most often as enemies. This relationship is a more conflictual one psychologically than the first one described. While it is generally possible for victims to feel anger at those responsible for their loss, there is also some tendency to internalize a sense of themselves as worthless, with acceptance of the notion that only worthless people would be targeted for destruction. Thus, survivors of the Hiroshima bombing tend to hold feelings of worthlessness throughout their lives. In a curious twist, Lifton found that some Hiroshima survivors blamed their own government for not protecting them, rather than the Americans, whom they held in awe for the "greatness" of their weapon (Lifton, 1967).

c. In the third and most psychologically complex relationship, the victim group is in some way dependent upon the agents of the disaster. This dependence is usually an economic one, as it is at Three Mile Island, Love Canal, and Buffalo Creek. In the latter two cases, the entire region is directly or indirectly dependent on the chemical or coal industry for economic survival. The psychological impact of the victims' experience of impotence in relation to a company or industry which provides their livelihood but which is killing them is enormous. In an exploitative work relation, people tend to internalize views of themselves as worth no more than what they produce and to see themselves not only as less powerful, but also as inferior to those for whom they produce. This self-view is exaggerated in a disaster which results from the priority of profit over human life.

Lifton and Olson (1976) describe the people of Buffalo Creek as continuing in a state of "bitter resentment and unrelieved dependency" which is a powerful force leading to self-hatred rather than activism. They found that even though survivors experienced rage toward the company for the loss of loved ones and homes, the internalization of worthlessness and the feelings of powerlessness prevented the expression of, or constructive acting on, that anger. Two factors may be at work here. Psychologically, the experience of helpless rage over harm or abandonment by the source of sustenance and power evokes the most frightening and paralyzing aspects of infantile experience. A defensive solution used in infancy may then be called up—experiencing self, rather than the powerful other, as bad. Many concentration camp victims, who were totally dependent on their unrelentingly brutal captors for each day of survival, internalized the Nazi view of themselves as worthless and bad to the point that they no longer believed that they *deserved* to live (Krystal, 1968).

On a socioeconomic level, in a capitalist society it is very difficult to find acceptable targets for rage in a disaster situation. Is it the fault of the coal company foreman (who is known to people but does not make the decisions), the president of the individual coal company, the coal industry, or the economic system that places profit before life? In our depoliticized society, the last two choices are rarely considered, and the preceding ones seem too personal: the psychological result is that victims do not find suitable targets for their anger and so cannot reach resolution.

Preexisting Psychological Functioning of the Individual Victim

Generally speaking, the ability to master a traumatic situation without serious long-term impairment is related to the degree of unresolved emotional conflict prior to the trauma and the extent to which the content of the trauma feeds into preexisting conflict (Lindemann, 1944; Wolfenstein, 1957; Kliman, 1968). This generalization seems to hold for the trauma of a disaster situation as well. As mentioned earlier, however, the literature on the Holocaust suggests that experience with chronic, brutal and pervasive death and humiliation is overwhelming to the point that it can lead to psychopathology regardless of prior level of functioning.

Earlier in this chapter, we discussed evidence that people who defend against their frightening hostile impulses by projecting them onto others tend to perceive the disaster as punishment more than other victims. Since punishment was not completed (i.e., the victim did not perish) and the survivor experienced relief that it was others who died instead, there is likely to be continuing anxiety about the recurrence of the disaster punishment. On the other hand, those who defend against both their angry impulses and their feelings of vulnerability by denying the possibility of danger from or to oneself are more likely to have their defensive systems shattered and to be left emotionally devastated by the disaster. These two groups are among those Wolfenstein (1957) found most at risk in the wake of disaster. People who had previously experienced an inadequately resolved loss antecedent to the catastrophe and who tend to attach the disaster experience onto prior conflict would also be predisposed to develop dysfunctional means of coping with the feelings of abandonment and loss generated by the disaster (Kliman, 1968).

Wolfenstein points to a particular risk for characterologically depressed individuals after a disaster. She states that "normal" people in a disaster experience a transient reactive depression, which is often followed by the also transient elation during the postdisaster utopia.

The ability to turn passive experience into an active mastery is crucial to the effective resolution of the disaster trauma, in that it allows for a greater control over one's situation and one's fate. Several variables are involved in the ability to master the trauma. One is prior psychologically "immunizing" experiences with less overwhelming situations of loss or fear (Kliman, 1968). Another is having a role which allows one to be responsible and active, rather than being a passive recipient: being helpful to others is psychologically helpful to oneself in times of severe stress.

One of the most powerful ways to effect psychological mastery of a disaster is to take an activist position in the community in the period following the disaster. This activism can take several forms. Participation in rescue and reconstruction work allows victims to "undo" some of the damage done to their social and physical environment. Working with community pressure groups and other formal and informal organizations to ensure adequate care and compensation for disaster victims, or increased protection against potential future disasters is useful psychologically as well as politically. A third possibility is found in political and educational work, for instance, concerning the risks entailed in nuclear energy, or organized attempts to shut down or better safeguard power plants, in the case of victims of the Three Mile Island accident.

Outlets for the feeling and expression of distress are crucial to the ability to master the disaster situation. In Corning and Xenia, Kliman (1976) found that people who were able to talk about their fear, anger, frustration, depression, and confusion, and share those feelings with others, were less likely to exhibit psychological symptoms in the long run. Significant differences were found between the anxiety levels of those children who were encouraged to talk in school about the disaster and their responses to it and those who did not have that opportunity. It is unfortunate that in American culture, there is a prevailing belief in the value of quiet, uncomplaining strength, in keeping a "stiff upper lip" and not burdening others with our problems. This attitude is not conducive to master of trauma, but rather to suppression of psychological conflict.

There is a relationship between individuals' belief systems and their psychological functioning following a disaster. Wolfenstein (1957) suggests that Jewish religious beliefs, which allow for the possibility that God might punish without withdrawing love, may have been helpful in mitigating the sense of total abandonment experienced by European Jews during the Holocaust. Such a belief might be somewhat soothing in the event of a more "normal" disaster as well. Lifton (1967) also found that religious and political beliefs had an impact on the ability of Hiroshima survivors to resolve their experience of the atomic bombing. In fact, his work suggests that any belief system which provides a framework into which the disaster experience can be integrated may be very helpful in the process of resolution and mastery. For example, Marxist and other leftist survivors had political explanations of the bombing and its aftermath that provided clear channels for anger (against the ruling classes of all countries, including the United States and Japan), and a sense of responsibility for acting on their understanding of the event. These survivors were somewhat better equipped to reach resolution of their traumatic experience than people without such a comprehensive and activism-oriented belief system (Lifton, 1967).

Direct, Indirect, and Hidden Victims of Disaster

Victims' social and psychological experiences of disaster vary considerably in connection with the form their victimization takes. Direct victims, those who have suffered loss or injury, tend to experience feelings and symptoms of depression, which are related to the loss and abandonment encountered in the disaster, and of anxiety, which is related to guilt at surviving while others did not, and fear of not surviving the next disaster. Indirect victims, on the other hand, are more likely to experience guilt and stress-related symptoms, such as accidents, fights, and disease-involving hypertension (Kliman, 1976). While direct victims are the worst affected by a disaster, in our society they are also the only victims whose suffering is given credence. Some validation is received for the feelings of despair and loss and more social and emotional help is willingly provided to direct victims.

For the indirect victim, the picture is not as clear-cut. Nothing has actually "happened" to the individual him/herself, so all the intense feelings and psychosomatic, stress-related symptoms that emerge in the weeks or months following the disaster are confusing. People cannot understand why they are so irritable, achey and unable to concentrate. The fact is, of course, that something *has* happened to them. Their community has been damaged. People in their social networks have been killed, hurt, or left homeless. Their whole social world has been turned upside down. In addition, a powerful sense of "there but for the grace of God go I," and a fear that next time they will not be personally safe can be extremely anxiety- and guilt-provoking. Finally, for the indirect victim, who has had to confront his/her own mortality in the course of the disaster, the special attention and concern given to the direct victims, while indirect victims are ignored, can lead to a resentment which further intensifies guilt feelings.

The psychological functioning of the caregivers, who are the *hidden victims* of a disaster, is usually overlooked in disaster research and intervention. They are called hidden victims because, unless they are also members of the stricken community (in which case they are also direct or indirect victims), they were in no way part of the initial disaster experience. They were not subjected to the initial terror, loss, or abandonment that other victims were. However, these are the people who do much of the rescue work, provide succor, and act as gatekeepers for financial and other forms of aid in the weeks and months following the disaster, and they cannot help but be emotionally affected by their contact with the disaster situation. The guilt experienced by indirect victims is also at work here since direct victims come to caregivers precisely *because* of their own victim status, which is made all the more vivid by virtue of the caregiver's relatively secure position.

The hidden victim must begin the process of psychic numbing if he/she is to be effective in working with direct or indirect victims, and this numbing is in itself guilt-inducing. Rescue workers often report suppressing with great effort their painful responses to dead or badly injured bodies so they can continue with their essential work. When the numbing wears off, however, caregivers often get disgusted with themselves for being "callous." Like the direct victim, the hidden victim needs to know that there are good reasons for the emotional distress experienced in disaster, even when one's own family and home are intact.

Class and Gender Position

Class position temporarily loses its salience in the immediacy of catastrophe, as most disasters are indiscriminate in the havoc they wreak. In fact, the early (downward) leveling effects of disaster often contribute to an initial sense of egalitarianism and of a community of suffering among all segments of the stricken population. These effects do not continue very far into the reconstruction period.

Earlier in the chapter, we described the process through which the predisaster political *status quo* is legitimated and reestablished, after a brief period in which many decisions are shared and consensual. This return to political "business as usual" is legitimated in part through the official manipulation of information and explanations regarding the disaster, its management, and aftermath. Much as political decisions are shared during the emergency, so are economic resources, in a generosity born of a shared experience transcending class, race, and other usually divisive lines. This momentary and context-specific "socialism" cannot be maintained for any length of time within the large capitalistic system, however, and as the immediate emergency passes, there is a return to the original unequal distribution of wealth and resources.

After a time when tragedy and resources were both shared on a more equitable level than usual, a return to the old economic order must be legitimated if those who stand to gain most by maintaining the emergency social system and to lose most by returning to the original system are to be kept quiescent.

For members of the lower classes, the realization that the economic equalization that the "postdisaster utopia" promised was illusory, coupled with strong official criticism of attempts to gain from postdisaster economic relief, promotes the tendency to experience disaster as punishment. The grief, guilt, and anger engendered by the loss of loved ones knows no class boundaries. However, differences in the social and material conditions, which face people in different economic positions after the disaster, make for significant variations in the psychology of postdisaster life. Not only do working-class and poor people find themselves in greater financial difficulty than before the disaster, while they see members of the middle and upper classes recoup their temporary economic losses, they are also forced to contend with this inequity while they are in mourning for loved ones, homes, health, possessions, and stability. Under these circumstances, victims on the low end of the economic ladder are bound to feel both a decline in self-esteem (in part since they are unable to "pull themselves up by their own bootstraps") and resentment toward those who are more fortunate.

Class differences are also seen in the way people view official reports and explanations of the disaster and its aftermath. In both Three Mile Island and Love Canal, poor and working-class people were somewhat more likely to believe official communications underplaying the danger to which they were being exposed (Leaser, 1980; Maloney, 1980). This contrast may relate not only to differences in educational level, but also to the fact that people with fewer economic resources have fewer options to consider (e.g., moving) and may therefore be more likely to exercise denial in a defense against the painful awareness that they cannot keep themselves and their families safe. For example, a number of low-income housing project residents who live on the periphery of the contaminated section of Love Canal have been lobbying to buy up the homes of middle-income people the government has relocated, since those houses can now be had at extremely low prices. Denial of danger is essential to understanding such a decision. An additional explanation of the contrast is that working-class people are socialized toward a greater respect for authority (Kliman, 1979).

Gender also appears to play a role in the form that psychological reactions to disaster takes. Recalling Barton's (1970) findings on responses to the immediate emergency situation, we see that women are more likely than men to be dazed initially. Gender differences in long-term reactions to disaster may be more significant, however, gender plays its most important role in two areas of postdisaster functioning: (1) the development of psychological and psychogenic symptoms related to various kinds of emotional conflict, and (2) the ways in which the aftereffects of the disaster are perceived.

In the communities surrounding Three Mile Island, doctors have found that in the year following the nuclear accident, men complained of gastrointestinal distress such as nausea, vomiting, and diarrhea and of muscular aches and pains more frequently than women. Women, on the other hand, were more prone to hysterical symptomatology—even to the point of hysterical conversion paralysis and numbness (rare symptoms for this population) in a small number of cases. Leaser (1980) suggests, and we concur, that these differences in symptomatology relate to the effects of socialization to gender roles. In general, men are discouraged from expressing distress and fear, with the result that these feelings are likely to be manifested on a somatic level. It is considered more acceptable for women to verbalize these feelings, thus decreasing the need for such forms of somaticization. However, women are also socialized into feelings of helplessness in times of stress, as is manifested through hysterical symptoms and most dramatically through hysterical paralysis. Indeed, in the Three Mile Island area, women have been more verbally expressive of their anxiety, fear, and general upset in response to the accident and continuing dangers of radiation than men.

The fact that men and women perceive the ongoing dangers connected to the aftereffects of the accident differently is evident in the strong disagreements between many spouses as to the wisdom of staying in the Three Mile Island vicinity. Many more women than men have expressed the belief that moving away from the area is essential to the health of their families. Men, on the other hand, are far more likely to worry about the financial losses entailed in relocating, and to underplay the medical risks involved in staying. These opposing positions appear to contribute greatly to the increase in marital discord reported in the months since the accident. Leaser (1980), in reporting this information, hypothesizes that the gender difference relates to women, particularly in a blue-collar community, tending to be more familiar with, hence more realistic about, issues of family health and less familiar with and realistic about the economics of the job and housing markets. For men, the situation is reversed. Each group is liable to be overly optimistic about things working out for the best in the realm with which they are less familiar. We would add to this analysis that gender serves as a framework through which perceptions and expectations of the world are organized over the course of a lifetime. As these findings are preliminary and tentative, further research on the influence of gender on postdisaster experience should be carried out.

CONCLUSIONS AND IMPLICATIONS FOR CRISIS INTERVENTION

The focus of this chapter has been on some of the psychological implications of the relationship between various kinds of disasters and the communities and individuals they touch. We have argued that community and individual responses to disasters and their aftermaths can be understood and even predicted through an examination of the nature and social meaning of the particular disaster, the characteristics of the communities and individuals affected, and the form the relationship takes between the disaster and its victims.

A number of variables have been identified as important to the understanding of psychological reactions to disaster. Of these variables, several are particularly significant. The first four are "sociological" in nature and the last two are "psychological." They are: *(1)* the origin of the disaster (i.e., whether it is the result of human or natural activity); *(2)* the extent to which culpability can be attributed to agents of a human-made disaster (because the disaster was intentional or predictable); *(3)* the nature of the historical and continuing social, economic, and political relationship between the agents and victims of human-made disaster; *(4)* the extent to which the disaster's physical effects are limited in time; *(5)* whether victimization is direct, indirect or "hidden"; and *(6)* the victims' level of psychological functioning prior to the disaster.

Of the first four, "sociological" variables, we can say that it is harder to achieve psychological resolution and mastery of the losses incurred in human-made disaster than in natural disaster. When catastrophes are human in origin, this difficulty is greatly compounded if the disaster is also intentional or predictable, if disaster victims are in any way dependent on the agents of the disaster, or if the disaster effects continue through time. Psychological mastery is bound to be most difficult when all of these conditions hold true. These important differences must be taken into account in planning individual and community crisis interventions in the wake of disaster.

A dynamic interaction exists between the social variables discussed in this chapter and the psychological characteristics and needs of disaster victims. In order to make effective therapeutic interventions in the wake of disaster (or, for that matter, in order to be effective in any form of therapeutic relationship), it is essential that psychological functioning be placed in its social context. Mental health workers who provide therapeutic or consultative interventions in communities struck by disasters, whether caused by natural or human forces, must conceptualize the relationship between social and psychological conditions. It is equally important to develop a *practice* that is based on that conceptualization, addressing the social, economic and political realities in which psychological responses to disaster are imbedded. Intrinsic to this model of community crisis intervention is a view of mental health workers as facilitators of active collective as well as individual attempts at mastery of the disaster.

We know from the "psychological first aid" work provided to

individuals and communities in natural disasters that a number of strategies are of particular help in the facilitation of resolution of the disaster. The two most crucial therapeutic goals to be pursued in the weeks and months following a disaster, regardless of the circumstances of the disaster itself, are facilitating the expression of distress and the transformation of passive experience into active mastery.

Both of these goals can be attained through crisis intervention done with individuals, families, and therapy groups, and psychotherapy is advisable for people whose prior psychological functioning, severe victimization by the disaster, or other vulnerability suggests a high risk for the development of psychopathology following disaster. For the majority, however, these two goals can be attained, for primary preventive purposes, without resorting to formal therapeutic work. Kliman's (1976) work in Corning showed that the utilization of "town meetings," and of such "natural groups" as PTAs, neighborhood associations, children's classes, and the staff meetings of service organizations and businesses for sharing feelings about the disaster and its aftermath is quite helpful in reducing stress responses. Passive experience can be turned into active mastery through participation in community groups working toward reconstruction, lobbying government agencies, providing community education or relief work, and the strengthening of social networks as informal mutual support groups (Kliman, 1976). Both kinds of facilitative work help people to develop a sense of shared experience and ability which counters feelings of isolation, abandonment, and guilt, and decreases feelings of helplessness and low self-esteem.

These goals can also be attained through training caregivers, such as social workers, teachers, Red Cross volunteers, medical personnel, and others to be aware of disaster victims' needs to maintain a sense of autonomy and dignity at a time when they are most vulnerable and needy. In addition, when these caregivers, the hidden victims, are helped by mental health consultants to accept their own confusing and difficult feelings about the disaster and its victims, the victims themselves should be better able to express and accept their emotional responses to disaster and its aftermath.

We know a good deal about the strategies for crisis intervention that are most effective in helping individuals and communities deal with natural disasters (Kliman, 1976). Much less is known through experience about what kinds of intervention strategies are most helpful when disasters are wrought by people. Information has been accumulating over the last few years, however, about collective and individual responses to various kinds of human-made disaster. This information, much of which is presented in this chapter, helps to lay the groundwork for developing a paradigm of crisis intervention into human-made disaster.

REFERENCES

Barton, *Communities in Disaster: A Sociological Analysis of Collective Stress Situations.* Garden City: Anchor, 1970.

Bettelheim, B. *The Informed Heart.* Glencoe: The Free Press. 1963.

Brown, M. and Goldin, A. Collective Behavior: A Review and Reinterpretation of the Literature. 1979

Cowan, P. Harrisburg: Something in the Air. *The Village Voice,* 1980, *25*(12), March 24, 1980.

Dohrenwend, B. and Dohrenwend, B., eds. *Stressful Life Events: Their Nature and Effects.* New York: Wiley, 1974.

Erikson, K. *Everything in its Path: Destruction of Community in the Buffalo Creek Flood.* New York: Simon and Schuster, 1976.

Frankl, V. *From Death Camp to Existentialism.* New York: Beacon. 1959.

Franklin, B. A. Long Distress Found Over Atom Accident. *The New York Times,* April 18, 1980.

Kliman, A. "The Corning Flood Project: Psychological First Aid Following a Natural Disaster," in Parad, H., Resnick, H., and Parad, L., eds. *Emergency and Disaster Management: A Mental Health Sourcebook.* Bowie, Md.: Charles Press, 1976.

Kliman, A. *Crisis: Psychological First Aid for Recovery and Growth.* New York: Holt, Winston and Rhinehart, 1978.

Kliman, G. *Psychological Emergencies of Childhood.* New York: Grune and Stratton, 1968.

Kliman, J. Children and Authority: An Exploration in Political Socialization. Unpublished doctoral dissertation, The Wright Institute, Berkeley, 1979.

Krystal, H., ed. *Massive Psychic Trauma.* New York: International Universities Press, 1968.

Leaser, J. Personal communication, 1980.

Lifton, R. J. *Death in Life—Survivors of Hiroshima.* New York: Random House, 1967.

Lifton, R. J., and Olson, Eric. Death Imprint in Buffalo Creek, in Parad, H., Resnik, H., and Parad, L., eds. *Emergency and Disaster Management: A Mental Health Sourcebook.* Bowie, Md.: Charles Press, 1976.

Lindemann, E. Symptomatology and Management of Acute Grief. *American Journal of Psychiatry,* 1944, 101, 141–148

Luchterhand, E. G. Sociological Approaches to Massive Stress in Natural and Man-Made Disaster. *International Psychiatric Clinics,* 1971, *8*, 29.

Maloney, J. Personal communication, 1980.

Niederland, W. The Psychiatric Evaluation of Emotional Disorders in Survivors of Nazi Persecution, in Krystal, H., ed. *Massive Psychic Trauma.* New York: International Universities Press, 1968.

Schiller, H. *The Mind Managers.* New York: Beacon Press, 1973.

Speck, R. and Attneave, C. *Family Networks.* New York: Pantheon, 1973.

Sterba, Edith. The Effects of Persecution on Adolescents, in Krystal, H., ed. *Massive Psychic Trauma.* New York: International Universities Press, 1968.

Timkoe, G. Personal communication, 1980.

Wolfenstein, M. *Disaster: A Psychological Study.* Glencoe: Free Press, 1957.

Zusman, J. Meeting Mental Health Needs in a Disaster: A Public Health View, in Parad, H., Resnik, H., and Parad, L., eds. *Emergency and Disaster Management: A Mental Health Sourcebook.* Bowie, Md.: Charles Press, 1976.

INDEX